Caring for Your Masterpiece

Health from a Biblical, Real Food point of view

By Mrs. Betty Tracy

Drink more water
Eat more veggies
Get more exercise
Love God and His People

This is the path to health

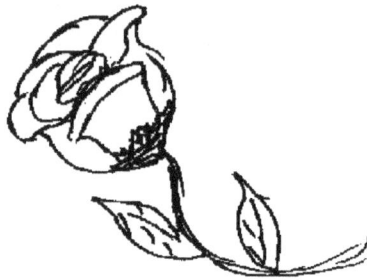

"Thou shalt not muzzle the ox that treadeth out the corn. And, the laborer is worthy of his reward." 1 Timothy 5:18 (1 Corinthians 9:9, Deuteronomy 25:4, Luke 10:7, Matthew 10:10, Deuteronomy 24:15.)

"Therefore, behold, I am against the prophets, saith the Lord, that steal my words every one from his neighbor." Jeremiah 23:30

:...Thou shalt not steal, ... Thou shalt love thy neighbor as thyself." Romans 13:9 (Matthew 19:18, Mark 10:19, Luke 18:20, 1 Corinthians 6:8,10, Ephesians 4:28, Exodus 20:15, Leviticus 19:11,13, Deuteronomy 5:19, Leviticus 19:18, Matthew 5:43, 7:12, 19:19, 22:39, Mark 12:31, Luke 10:27, Galatians 5:14, James 2:8)

"Render therefore to all their dues: ... honor to whom honor." Romans 13:7

"That no man go beyond and defraud his brother in any matter: because that the Lord is the avenger of all such, as we also have forewarned you and testified." 1 Thessalonians 4:6 (Leviticus 19:13, Deuteronomy 32:35, Proverbs 22:22,23) Scriptures compiled by the Bluedorns, Triviumpursuit.com.

Table of Contents

1. A Masterpiece of the Master Artist

Philosophy, Wisdom, and Definitions

"Before I formed thee in the belly I knew thee, and before thou came out of the womb I sanctified thee."
Jeremiah 1:5

You are a Masterpiece of Art created by The Master Artist. Your body may not be what you think of as beautiful, but to God it is. Your magnificent body was given to you as a special gift. Think of how wondrously God created you; from your thumbs to your eyeball, you are a triumph of Divine engineering.

The best way to show someone that you are thankful for a gift given to you is to take care of that gift and use it properly. There are many ways to care for our bodies.

My Basic Philosophy on Health.

I believe God created us. We are not a series of accidents, but the deliberate design of an all knowing, loving God. He provided us with everything we need to be perfectly healthy and happy and to live forever.

The first man, Adam, sinned and brought the curse of death on the whole universe. Because of this, we get sick and will eventually die. Life is fatal. No matter what we do, we won't get out of it alive. This is a fact.

But the better we take care of our bodies, the better we will feel and the more we can accomplish for God before we die. This doesn't mean we won't be sick. We still live under the curse and in a fallen world. It just means we lower our chances and severity of illness, at least until our final illness.

We must work at maintaining our health, but this is the least we can do to show God how thankful we are for this wondrous gift of life.

"And God said, Behold, I have given you every herb bearing seed, which is upon the face of all the earth, and every tree, in which is the fruit of a tree yielding seed; to you it shall be for food."
Genesis 1:29

Right after creating humankind, God told them they could eat of any of the plants and trees in the garden. In fact, because death came with Adam's sin, they would have been vegetarians before the Fall. That means the plants and trees in the garden contained everything necessary to life.

"And unto Adam He said, '…cursed is the ground for thy sake. In sorrow shall thou eat of it all the days of thy life. Thorns also and thistles shall it bring forth to thee, and thou shall eat the herb of the field. In the sweat of thy face shall thou eat bread, till thou return unto the ground.' " Genesis 3:17-19

After the fall, man was to eat not just the plants and trees, but God instructed them to eat bread also (herb of the field), and the very dirt is cursed. I believe this means our dirt is dying and not as productive as it used to be.

"Every moving thing that lives shall be food for you, just like the green herb have I given you all things." Genesis 9:3

After the flood, God told Noah he could eat meat- the flesh of animals. I have no proof, but I think something in the flood changed the dirt of our planet enough that life could no longer be easily supported without adding meat to the diet. God knew this was going to happen and gave us meat-eating teeth and a meat-eater's apendix at Creation, as well as a meat-eater's instincts. We are equipped to handle flesh better, in fact, than plants. Plant eaters have much larger appendixes in order to better digest the plant matter.

When God gave the Mosaic Law He gave ceremonial, moral/civic, and health laws. They were all symbolic of Christ and the church. None of them are important today for our salvation.

However, if we were to follow the moral/civic laws, our countries would be nicer places to live, (in fact, the American Founding Fathers based our original laws on the Mosaic Law).

If we follow the health laws, we would probably be healthier.

"There is a way which seems right unto a man, but the end of it are the ways of death."
Proverbs 14:12

Whenever man has tried to "improve" on anything God has done, he messes it up. There are negative consequences (usually unseen at first). The closer we can stay to the way God made things in the beginning, the healthier we will be.

Now, fixing what is broken due to the Fall is different. Man can repair bones, stop heart attacks and do all sorts of wonderful repair jobs. We should thank the Lord that we live in a time with this technology available.

But when it comes to improving on the original creation of God, man always messes it up somehow.

Let's take vaccinations for example. A vaccination is the injection of a (in most cases dead) disease-causing organism in order to trigger the immune system to build anti-bodies against the disease, making your body think you have had it before and so you don't get it again. This makes perfect sense, right? There are a few problems though:

Many vaccines wear off. We all know we need a Tetanus booster every ten years. Most do not know that the MMR (Measles, Mumps, Rubella) vaccine also wears off, giving the child immunity during the safest years for him to have the disease (childhood) and leaving him vulnerable during the most dangerous (childbearing) years. This is also true for other vaccines. Boosters are not currently available for these other vaccines.

They don't always work. "50% of all whooping cough cases are in those who are not fully vaccinated." This means that 50% of all whooping cough cases are in those who ARE fully vaccinated. Why put this disease and its poisonous preservatives into my child's body when it has so little affect on their risk for contracting the disease?

Some vaccines CAUSE the disease they are supposed to prevent. All cases of polio in the last thirty years in America, for example, have been caused by the vaccine (baby gets vaccinated, mommy changes baby's diaper, mommy contracts Polio. Live vaccines can shed the virus for as long as 2 weeks after the shots, meaning recently vaxed children are contagious.)

The first county in the world to be declared Small Pox free was a county in England that had not been vaccinating for it for 2 years. Everyone else, who were still vaccinating, still had the occasional case pop up.

Also, a woman who had measles in chilhood passes immunity to her baby as long as she is nursing, so babies (who are at risk for severe complications of Measles) don't get it. But a mom who never had Measles, only the vaccine, does not pass any immunity to Measles to her baby, leaving him at risk.

All medical procedures have some risk. For example, Thermosil (the preservative in the flu and some other vaccines) may be linked to Autism. The research is still ongoing, but there are too many stories of babies who are perfectly healthy until the day they get a shot, and then are autistic or otherwise damaged for me to believe the shots don't casue many problems, including autism.

Some children have bad immediate reactions to vaccines; fever, convulsions, deafness, death. You don't know if your child is one of them until AFTER they have the shots. Bad reactions are irreversible.

We don't really know what we are doing to our children's immune systems. The rates of allergies (mild as well as life threatening) have skyrocketed in the last sixty years. Some are saying we are not keeping our homes clean enough. Some say too clean. Some blame overhead power lines, preservatives in our foods, pesticides, plastic carpets, and all sorts of things. Could it really be something as simple as messing with a child's immune system through vaccinations? Allergies and asthma are immune responses. Are we damaging their immune system by giving them a vaccine to prevent an otherwise, usually mild disease (ear infection, chicken pox, measles, etc.)? I don't know, but this is actually the most logical explanation I have heard for the cause of the increase in asthma and allergies.

The manufacturers and the CDC don't even pretend they test vaccines for long term side affects (or affects on fertility and mutogenic properties), much less compare the over all health of the vaccinated with the over all health of the unvaccinated.

One recent study found that all diabetic children had a certain antibody to a protein in milk (Antibodies to disease are good. Antibodies to food are bad. Milk protein is a food). Pasteurization changes the proteins in milk. Could the change in the immune system caused by vaccinations be causing our own systems to attack this changed protein in pasteurized milk thus destroying our pancreases and causing Diabetes? It is known that those who receive the MMR vaccine have a higher rate of Diabetes than those who don't. This may just be an accidental correlation, but then again, it may not be. Today we are seeing epidemic rates of Diabetes (one out of every three people have it). We have a "fully vaccinated" population. Hmmmm.

But haven't vaccines saved lives?

Some, such as Small Pox and Tetanus, may have. However, the rates of comunicable diseases that there are vaccinations for declined by as much as 40% BEFORE vaccinations were available (vaccinations were not made available until roughly 1945, yet ALL communicable diseases saw a drastic decline starting in the early 1900's, including Scarlet Fever and Typhoid, which we still don't have vaccines for, yet have disappeared at the same rate as Measles and Mumps). This is due to improved sanitation (indoor plumbing), cleaner water, penicillin and better nutrition (making the immune system stronger and better able to fight disease). This means that the large decline of "childhood" diseases that is usually attributed to vaccinations could not possibly be because of the shots.

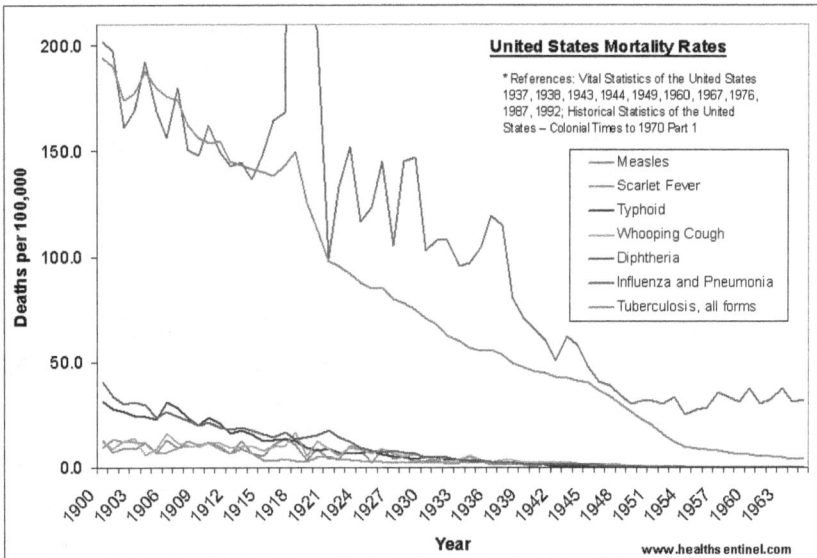

Our family evaluated the potential lifelong risks of the vaccines compared to the potential lifelong risks of the diseases they are supposed to prevent. We believe the vaccines carry a greater long-term risk of permanent damage (especially since diabetes and asthma run so high in my family). Our children are well fed and strong. Even if they contract one of these diseases, the chances of permanent damage are very low.

Even the Tetanus vaccine is suspect. Tetanus declined right along with all the other communicalbe diseases, even though it is not really a communicalbe disease.

Tetanus: mean annual death rates: England and Wales

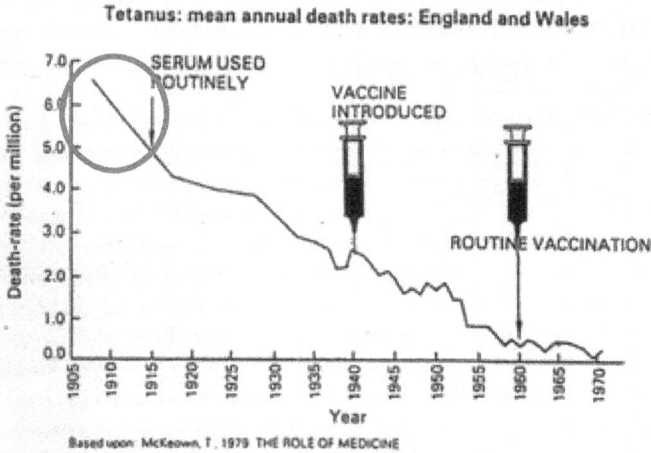

Figure 1adoseoftruth.weebly.com

The CDC recently discussed five children with Tetanus. Two were vaccinated and three weren't. None died. In fact, those who do die of this disease in America are almost universally elderly with diabetes. You see, the Tetanus virus will die if exposed to oxygen, so if any wound bleeds (blood carries oxygen) the virus will die. If mommy makes sure the wound is fully washed out too, there is no chance of the virus living much less growing. Diabetics have poor blood circulation so their wounds are less likely to bleed and kill the virus.

If you or your child does show signs of Tetanus, take them to the emergency room and ask for the Tetanus Immunoglobulin shot. Not the vaccine, the TiG. It will kill the virus in the system. I choose not to expose my children to the risks of the vaccine for a disease they are not likely to get and that can be cured with a shot if they do get it.

I believe every parent should do the research for themselves. Ask for and read the vaccine inserts (not just the papers they give out with the shots) in the doctor's office before you bring your child in, read the information on the CDC web site, read some of the "Don't Vaccinate" literature and web sites[1]. Google each disease. Certainly PRAY about it. Weigh the risks and benefits for YOUR family. They will be different than for mine.

Some more information:

Some vaccines are unnecessary for some children.

Hepatitis B is a disease contracted by gays, prostitutes, and IV durg users, those that work with them (doctors and nurses), babies of HepB moms, daycare children and daycare workers. This vaccine is routinly given to a child on the day he is born. If your newborn baby is not engaging in gay behavior, prostitution, taking drugs, treating these people in a medical situation (handling their blood), or in daycare they don't need this vaccine. If they decide to join a medical profession as an adult, or choose thse life styles, they can get the vaccine then.

Instead of injecting every baby with HepB, why don't we add a HepB blood test to all the other blood tests we run on moms birthing in hospitals? If mom is positive, by all means! Give that baby the vaccine! It wil save his life.

---

[1] Some good resources are Shonda Parker's "Mommy Diagnostics," "How to Have a Healthy Child In spite of Your Doctor," and "What Your Doctor May Not be Telling You About Vaccinations."

But if mom isn't positive, baby is not at risk of getting the disease. Why give him the shot?

The **HPV** vaccine (Guardasil) is for a type of cervical cancer transferred by promiscuous sexual behavior (it's an STD). The vaccine has been tested on older teen girls, not children, yet the recommendation is for all children of school age to receive it. We don't yet know the long term side effects, nor if the vaccine wears off. We do know that approximately three times as many young women are being permanently damaged or even killed by reactions to this vaccine than they expect to contract the cancer it is supposed to prevent! If your daughters are not engaging in sexual behavior, especially if they are still little children, refuse this vaccine. And if your child is a boy, don't even think of allowing this vaccine (they did one short term test injecting the vaccine into mouse testes and then began giving it to all boys. We have no idea what this vaccine will do to fertility in these boys when they grow up). There is no scientificly tested reason for it; only profits for the drug industry.

The growth medium used in some vaccines (at least the MMR and Chicken pox) is aborted human fetal cells. They only need one baby every twenty years or so to grow the whole nation's worth of vaccines, but not only is this immoral, it's just plain gross. (Added note: Sometime after writing this, evidence came out that it may not be the Thermosil causing the rise in Autism, but the aborted fetus cells! And what do you suppose the results are of putting, say, baby girl fetal cells in a boy? We have no way of knowing yet.)

Vaccine companies tell us they removed the Thermosil a mercury based preservative). However independent testing companies say it is still in the vaccines. What the pharmaceutical companies are actually doing is using the Thermosil and then filtering it out. Of course they can't get all of it. Children are still being exposed to way too much mercury. And no one is even addressing the other poisons in the shots (i.e aluminum, fomaldehyde).

We don't want to inject poison into our children's bodies (unless there is a VERY good reason). The preservatives in vaccines are known poisons: Thermosil (mercury), formaldehyde, aluminum, etc. The less of these substances we can expose our children to the healthier they will be. The amount of mercury they put into my oldest child's body over the first two years of her life was an FDA approved safe dose....for a 400 POUND MAN!!! And they are adding more shots every year.[2] I thank the Lord she hasn't had any apparent reactions!

(By the way, this is a good reason to not put your child in daycare. This parenting decision is removed from you there. They insist that all children be vaccinated. And the CDC has declared daycares to be the single biggest transmission point for disease in America. An outbreak of one of these diseases could permanently close a center.)

Then there are anti-bacterial soaps and wipes. These sound wonderfully useful. They kill bacteria and viruses on contact. Great, right? Not so fast. They don't kill all microbes. They leave the strongest bad guys, killing all good microbes and the weaker bad ones leaving no

---

[2] Vaccinations are a big money maker for the pharmaceutical companies. They are the ones pushing to have so many shots become mandatory. Europe mandates about a third as many shots as the American government does.

competition for the really bad ones. We may actually be causing worse illnesses by removing God's competition for food among these organisms. We are also denying ourselves the good guys that aid digestion. And it is possible our immune systems are weaker because of the lack of exercise from not dealing with minor organisms, leaving us even more vulnerable.

The best prevention of disease is simply frequent washing with plain 'ole soap and water; something God commanded Israel to do in the books of the Law.

Man has put together large institutions for the efficient care and upbringing of children. Frees mom from child raising and allows her to pursue her own interests, right? No. We now know that children are best educated at home from birth, as God designed. He made breastfeeding so the young'uns must stay close to mom and commanded Israel to homeschool.

"And these words, which I command thee this day, shall be in thine heart. And thou shall teach them diligently unto thy children, and shall talk about them when thou sit in thine house, and when thou walk on the road, and when thou lie down, and when thou get up." Deuteronomy 6:6-7

This slows down the spread of disease, provides the children with individual tutors who actually care about them, trains them in godly behavior, and forces the parents to live up to what they are teaching since the children are watching them every moment. Many studies today show that daycare children have far more mental, physical, and intellectual problems, and homeschooling is superior to any other method of education in every measure (except for running speed. Seems government school children can run faster. More practice running from bullies, maybe?). Man's idea of the factory school/childcare just doesn't work well.

Humans think it doesn't matter what "lifestyle" you live as long as you are happy. But come to find out, those in all types of "alternative lifestyles (homosexual[3], co-habitating, divorce, polygamy, "swinging") have shorter life spans and way more health problems. They suffer from depression far more often than those in traditional, healthy relationships. What makes sense to humanity (that a relationship is about love and entertainment) is not what God says makes sense (a relationship is about obeying God, mirroring His relationship with the church, and producing godly offspring). Those who choose God's way of doing things are happier, healthier and have a longer life span on average.

---

[3] There is no scientific proof for the theory of homosexuality being caused by genetics. The few studies that have been done were incredibly poor science. For example, you need 1500 people to have a statistically reliable number for any study. The closer you have to 1500, the more likely you have the correct answer. The most reliable of all the studies that supposedly proved a "gay gene" had a whole sixteen participants. Autopsies were done on the brains of these men, some of whom claimed to be gay and some straight. The gay men had differences in their brains. Seems to prove the point doesn't it? But wait a minute, a few of the men who claimed to be straight (and did not have the different brain structure) died of AIDS. It is so close to impossible for a man to contract this disease from a woman, and since none of the participants were drug users, these men had to be closet gays. Also, it has been shown that psychoanalysis alone can change the composition of the brain. This means that what a person chooses to think changes the composition of their brain, not the other way around. The brain difference in the gays is the RESULT of their lifestyle choice, not the cause. Homosexuality is a choice, or more accurately, a series of choices.

Mankind thought it great to x-ray unborn babies to check their size and position. These children came down with Leukemia at much higher rates. (This makes some a little scared of Ultra-sounds. That technology has not really been around very long. We don't really know what long term affects it will have. Some evidence is beginning to look like frequent sonograms for no apparent reason might not be a good idea).

Mankind thought it wise to give women DES to prevent miscarriage. This caused baby girls to be born with messed up, duplicated, or no reproductive organs.

Man thought it best to give mommies with morning sickness Thalidomide to stop nausea. Their babies were born without arms and legs.

Man thinks it great to use Cytotec to induce labor. These births have a much higher rate of uterine rupture (potentially fatal to both mom and baby) and the contractions hurt a lot more putting baby at greater risk from pain killers.

I can go on and on with examples of how mankind has thought he has improved pregnancy and childbirth and child raising only to discover he has destroyed lives.

Can I give one more example? Mankind says to have your babies in hospitals. It is "more sanitary" and you have all those neat gadgets available in case of problems. Mankind has come to think of birth as an emergency medical procedure.[4]

---

[4] The US C-section rate is now 32%. The World Health Organization says no

Turns out though, hospitals aren't more sanitary. They are where sick people go. In fact, there are diseases that don't exist anywhere else on earth but in hospitals. Infection rates are much lower in homebirths. And all those gadgets being so handy make it way too easy to use them and mess up a perfectly natural process that God designed. Sometimes interventions are necessary (due to the Fall), but most of the time (90+%) they are not. God really did remember to tell a woman's body how to know when to start labor, to make her body big enough to birth a baby, and to give her the strength and fortitude to handle the pain (which Americans rate higher than anyone who doesn't have TV rates it). Many studies have shown that the place a woman's God-given instinct tells her is safest- her home- really is the safest place to have her baby. Mommy is already immune to the germs and mommy's body functions best away from the fear and stress of the hospital, in the place she feels most comfortable.

Now, though I do believe we should live as close to the original Creation plan as possible, there are very few, if any of us who actually can. I certainly don't measure up. The standards I set forth here are goals to reach for. I have not hit these yet myself. I am not even close in some areas. I am sharing what my research has me aiming for, not what I have accomplished.

---

country should have a rate higher than 10% and 5% is better. More than that is unnecessarily putting women at risk form this major abdominal surgery. See http://www.ican-online.org/

A Few Definitions for Nutrition

"My people are destroyed for lack of knowledge." Hosea 4:6

We have all heard many nutrition terms floating around. I thought it might be a good place to start by defining some of them.

Energy for cars is measured in miles-per-gallon. Energy for your lights is measured in kilowatt hours. Energy for your body is measured in **CALORIES**. A calorie is the amount of energy it takes to raise one centiliter of water one degree Celsius. There are four sources for calories; carbohydrates, protein, fats and alcohol.

A **GRAM** is the weight of water in one square centimeter (A square centimeter is about half the size of the last joint of your pinky).

CARBOHYDRATES and **PROTEINS** have four calories per gram.

FAT has nine calories per gram, and

ALCOHOL has seven calories per gram.

Each kind of energy source is used differently by the body.

CARBOHYDRATES are fuel for the muscles. Your body turns carbs into energy quickly and efficiently to use to make you go. There are two different kinds of carbs, simple and complex.

Simple carbs have a simpler molecular structure, while the complex carbs are, uhh, more complex (more atoms per molecule arranged in a more complex pattern.) The simple carbs digest almost instantly giving you a fast energy boost, but run out just as quickly, leaving you feeling kind of like you are riding a roller coaster; up and down, up and down.

Complex carbs take longer to digest, but longer to run out, also, and give a more even energy level.

Simple carbs are sugar, honey (though it digests slower than sugar), all syrups, and fruit juices.

Complex carbs are whole fruits, vegetables, breads, grains, cereals, and legumes (beans). Beans belong in both the carb and protein groups.

If you eat more carbs than your body uses within a couple of hours, your body will convert them into fat to save for later (fat saved in bubbles on the hips and thighs is often called cellulite. It is no different chemically than any other fat, just uglier and more noticeable).

FAT is used directly by the body to run the brain and can be converted into muscle energy. Fat digests slowly, coating your stomach making you feel fuller faster.

PROTEIN can be transferred into either muscle or brain fuel easily, so if you feel down and eat some protein you will get the boost where you are needing it most, whether in your muscles or your brain. Proteins are also used to build muscles, so if you exercise you need to eat protein to get the full effect.

FIBER comes in two forms; soluble and insoluble. Neither actually has calories, though they accompany unrefined carb calories (but not protein or fat). The soluble ones dissolve in your tummy and are absorbed by your blood and carried throughout your system. They act like a broom or scrub brush cleaning out your arteries. Insoluble fibers don't dissolve in your tummy. They go straight through, which is a very good thing because they act like brooms in your intestines pulling waste products out with them.

Those who eat diets high in both kinds of fiber have less digestive diseases (constipation, Irritable Bowl Syndrome, Colon Cancer, Diverticulitis) and less heart disease and Diabetes.

Refined carbs (white flour, white rice, all simple carbs) have had the fiber removed or never had any in the first place. If you want to see what they do to your intestines, just take a slice of white bread and get it wet. See how gooey and pasty it is? That stays in your intestines unless some fiber comes along and sweeps it out.

METABOLISM is the rate your body burns fuels (the equivalent of miles-per-gallon in your car). Some of us unlucky people have very efficient metabolisms. Our bodies need very little fuel to run on, yet our appetites and nutritional needs are as big as anyone else's. Dieting (starving) slows our metabolism down even more (a God designed mechanism to keep people from starving to death in a famine). Exercising speeds it up.

STRESS is the condition of the body produced by the "Fight or Flight" reflex. Americans live a high stress lifestyle. We are in a constant state of high alert, ready to "conquer the enemy." Unfortunately, this constant stress wears our systems out making us sick and vulnerable to disease.

VITAMINS are organic compounds required in tiny amounts by our bodies. The word vitamin is derived from the Latin "vita" which means "to live." They were available solely from food until just very recently. They were given an alphabet letter as well as a scientific name (Thiamin is vitamin B1 for example) when discovered. We manufacture some vitamins in our own system and some we must ingest.

MINERALS are inorganic compounds required by our bodies. They occur naturally in our dirt and are transferred to us through the foods we eat. We can also take supplements now.

(See the appendix for details on each vitamin and mineral.)

2. Mental Health

I am more and more convinced that this is the key issue in over-all health. Let's look at a well known fact: 40% of the time, a placebo will cure disease, (whether depression, headaches, hair loss, or even cancer.)

A **PLACEBO** is a medication made of totally inert, non-medicinal material ("sugar pill"). In order to see if new medications work, researchers will divide a group of people into two groups; the control group and the test group. The control group is given a placebo and the test group is given the new medicine (well done studies are careful to make the two groups as identical as possible and total as many people as possible). Neither the patients nor those dispensing the "medicines" know who is in which group. The new medicine is considered effective only if the test group has more "cures" than the control group. It is only safe if it has fewer side effects.[5]

This is how powerful the human brain is; it can cure itself of even cancer if it just thinks the body is supposed to get better.

If the brain can do this, then it can also make the body sick. So, I have put together a list of things you can do to make sure your brain is healthy, and thus your body.

1) **Believe in God.** Those who believe in a Divine Authority are healthier and recover from illness faster than those who don't. Having a belief in God means

---

[5] More recent studies sugest this format of study may even be unreliable. It seems they have discovered that those in the "medicine" group can figure out they are getting the medicine instead of the placebo by the sideaffects. Thus their brains kick into high gear since they "know" they should be getting well. This totally nullifies the results!

that you know Someone is in charge and there is ultimate justice. This lowers your stress levels and lets you believe there is a purpose in all things. It is a big weight off of our shoulders when we realize we are not personally responsible to run the world nor do we have to depend on those, ummm, "less than noble" people running this country and planet. We can trust that it will all work out in the end.

2) **Accept that you are a sinner.** You are not perfect. You will make mistakes and bad decisions. Knowing this allows you to relax and not take life so seriously. Other people are sinners and will make mistakes, too. Sometimes they will even hurt us. Forgive them for being imperfect, too. We are really no different than they are. We are all fallible. As one person put it "Take life seriously, but not too seriously." Or as my hubby says "Don't take life so seriously. You'll never get out of it alive."

3) **Accept Jesus as your Lord and Savior.** Since there is a God, and we are sinners, and sin separates us from God, we know that we need the price of our sins paid for us. We can never pay that price ourselves. Jesus paid that debt on Calvary for us. Accepting this puts us in His service and lets Him control our lives. It makes many of our decisions for us, reducing stress.

4) **Obey Christ's two commandments- "Love the Lord your God with all your heart, soul, mind and strength" and "Love your neighbor as yourself."** Doing this gives structure and guidance to your life. It makes most of your decisions for you, lowering your stress levels. It also causes you to be surrounded by

friends and family which leads to a longer, healthier, happier life.

5) **Choose to be thankful.** Thankful people don't wear themselves out pursuing what they don't need. They are content.

6) **Read your Bible Daily.** The Bible tells us about God. It is His love letter to us. The more we focus on His Word, the more peace we will have in our hearts and the more we will understand what His will is in our lives.

7) **Set goals for your life.** This gives you a reason to get up everyday and to feel good.

8) **Speak positively.** The Bible says;

"Because what he thinks in his heart, so is he..." Proverbs 23:7

When you hear negative thoughts coming out of your own mouth it reinforces them and makes you a negative person. Positive thoughts and words make you a positive person. Illness is negative; health is positive.

9) **Imagine yourself happy and healthy.** When you picture yourself, do you see a grumpy person or a smiling happy person? A sicky or a strong and healthy person? This is going back to the placebo effect. Thinking of yourself as healthy and happy will keep you healthier and happier.

10) **Keeping a journal** will help you to picture yourself happy and healthy and will help you work through those things that crop up to interfere with this thought pattern. People who begin to keep journals have reduced cases of asthma and other chronic disorders.

11) **Smile, hug, dance, laugh, play.** Choosing to do these things every day, even when you don't feel like

it, will make you healthier inside and out. Smile all the time (it reduces stress), hug at least three people everyday (also a stress reducer), dance at least once per day (good exercise and stress reducer), laugh for a minimum of ten minutes (produces endorphins; natures painkillers), and play often (for married couples this includes frequent sex. Orgasm produces hormones that physically and emotionally strengthen the heart.)

12) **Get plenty of exercise and sunshine.** I will cover exercise in its own section later.

God made us to spend time in the sunshine. Skin cancer is only caused by sunshine if you are deficient in vitamin A. It really doesn't make sense that an all knowing, all loving God would create something as all pervasive as sunshine that would harm us. I cover how to get plenty of vitamin A in the appendix.

Sunshine causes our skin to manufacture vitamin D; a necessary vitamin to bone formation. It also causes our skin to make serotonin, the anti-depression chemical, and is increasingly being shown to boost the immune system. We need plenty of God's sunshine (at least an hour per day) in order to be mentally healthy and strong.

Don't start off with an hour though. Start with fifteen minutes in the gentle light of the morning and work your way up. Expose as much of your body to the light as you can.

13) **Be quiet.** We are inundated with noise in our society. Right now sitting at my computer I hear its buzz, the dryer running, the fish tank's air pump, the answer machine (a "commercial" calling), cars on the road, and on and on (and I live in the country!) Some

of the noises we hear are so quiet we don't really notice them and others are quite loud. This constant stream of unnatural sounds distracts us and causes fatigue. Several times a week you should go somewhere where you can hear nothing manmade (birds and natural running water don't count as noise).

I also believe we need to take regular media fasts; times when we have no music playing, no TV on, no news, no cell phones, etc. So many in our world today fill their heads up with these things until they don't even know how to think for themselves. They are just used to having someone else fill their heads. I am beginning to wonder if most of us aren't afraid of our own thoughts! I think you should take at least half an hour every day to just be quiet and let God speak to your brain and listen to your own thoughts.

I also believe it is good to take time at least once per year (once per week would be better) to take a complete fast from all media. Don't read the paper, watch TV, listen to the radio, surf the net, or turn music on. Let your brain have a break. These fasts should last from a day (once per week) to at least a week (once per year). News, talk shows, fast or "cheating" music produce stress which encourages disease. We need time off occasionally from these things

14.   **Listen to positive music.** Fast paced music increases adrenalin and causes our bodies to function like they are in danger all the time. "Classical" (Artistic) music is the best for calming nerves and lowering adrenalin. Also, the Bible says, "whatsoever a man thinks, so is he." If you are listening to music talking about cheating on your spouse or killing people or in

any other way behaving in an ungodly manner, you will be desensitized to these behaviors and more tolerant of them. These behaviors (even just the thoughts) move you farther from the first four steps to health listed above.

15. **Get a pet and plant a garden.** God made us to be connected to His creation. Pets have been shown to reduce blood pressure and reduce stress. Gardens do the same. Both provide opurtunities for exercise. The more connection we have with God's creation the more we can come to understand Him and the more naturally our bodies will function. Remember, when God was done creating humans, He called them "Very Good" not "Very diseased."

16. **Eliminate debt.** Debt is one of the biggest stress-causers in our country. Did you know that if you just pay the minimum on your credit cards you will NEVER pay them off? The companies make their living by you paying interest. The longer you are a slave to them (**"The rich rules over the poor, and the borrower is servant to the lender."** Proverbs 22:7) the more money they make. So they keep your payments low enough to never completely pay the debt off. By eliminating all debt, you free yourself from this slavery.

The best way I have found to do this is to make a list of all your debts, how much you owe, and at what interest. Then pick the one you can pay off the fastest (even if it is the $20 you borrowed from Aunt Trudy) and work to pay it off. Make minimum payments to the others until you have the first paid off, putting every spare dime on it. Then take what you were paying to the first debt and apply it to the remaining one you can pay off the fastest.

When it is done, go to the next one, and so forth. This employs the snowball effect and really lets you feel like you are making headway quickly giving you the momentum needed to succeed.

Everyone has a budget (spending plan). The problem most people have is that they let the plan control them instead of the other way around. It is less stressful to control your spending plan with ways to meet your goals than to just let spending happen.

Make a list of all your income and all your expenses. Be sure to include giving to God. He has promised that if we take care of His work, He will take care of us. The general standard is 10%.

When you get paid, pay God first and you second. *Pay me?* Yes. Put a certain amount (aim for 10% if you possibly can) into savings. It is that money in savings that will keep you from going into further debt. Many try to have enough money in the bank that they could replace a major appliance, make repairs on the house or car, or pay medical bills if they need to with cash. They also pay their cars off and then keep making car payments to their own savings account, earning interest, with the goal of saving enough to pay cash for their next car. Over all, financial experts say the best plan is to have six months worth of expenses in the bank. That will cover most, if not all, potential emergencies without relying on credit cards.

Many Americans get themselves into financial trouble (financial illness) by overspending on housing and transportation (the two most common soft spots in people's hearts and heads). When you go to a bank to see how big of a loan you can get, they will try to give you as much money as possible because they make their living off the interest from your loan; the bigger the loan, the more interest. You must take responsibility for your own financial health as much as for your physical health, and not rely on others to tell you what you can handle.

Christian financial advisor Larry Burkett advised couples to figure how much housing they could afford as 40% of the HUSBAND'S income. What many young couples do is buy a house based on both their incomes and then get pregnant. This presents problems because now they have to choose between losing their home or giving baby the best care possible (mommy care). Basing your house price on the husband's income gives you the leeway to handle illness or children without too much stress. In the meantime, the wife's income can go to pay debts down (including the mortgage), and adding to the savings account.

"Housing" includes rent/mortgage, utilities, insurance, repairs, maintenance, and improvements. All this should, in most families, be about 40% of the hubby's income.

"Transportation" includes car payments, gas, insurance, DMV fees, tires, tune-ups, and bus fees. Transportation should come to around 10-15% of your income.

Food should be 10-20% (these numbers will be different for each family. For example, my hubby and I bought a house in foreclosure and spend way less than 40% on housing. However, with nine children, we spend way more than 20% on food. In fact, we spend more on food than housing. This is normal for our size family.) Food includes what you buy at the grocery store plus convenience foods (fast food, pizza) you buy because you are too tired or too busy to cook. It does not include the cost of dinner on mom and dad's date night, or the cost of lunch when the whole family goes to the fair. Those are entertainment expenses.

Here is a break down of the percentages for each category from the book "Financially Challenged" (after taxes, tithes, and saving 10%:

Housing- 35%

Transportation- 12%

Food- 11%

Insurance- 5%

Debt- 5%

Entertainment- 6%

Clothes- 5%

Medical- 12%

School/childcare- 6%

Miscellaneous (including Christmas and birthdays)- 2%

Surplus- 1%

Remember, if you spend more in one category than is listed, you have to spend less in another (as my family spends more on food but less on housing and transportation). Your total must add up to 100% or less or you have "Cancer Of The Budget."

(You figure percentage by dividing your income into the amount you spend in a category. For example, if your net income is $40,000 and you spend $5000 a year on daycare [$100/week], daycare is 12.5% of your income.)

One successful way to keep yourself on budget is called "The Envelope Method." You get one envelope for each category and divide your money into the appropriate place every payday. If you spend all that there is in one envelope, you are done with that category for the month. If you need to, you can borrow from another envelope, but then it shorts that category.

Of course, most of us spend plastic and don't actually use cash making this a little more difficult. The way to use this method when you don't use cash is to have a record page for each category, add the amount to spend in each category at each payday and subtract every time you spend. Or you can get free online bank accounts/pre loaded credit cards and assign one to each category (Akimbocard.com offers a pre-loaded mastercard with 5 sub-cards that can be named after your spending categories. So, I have a Christmas Tracy card and a Savings Tracy card, as well as separate cards for each of my minor children to put their allowances on.)

Finances are a major source of stress and thus physical illness. If you get yourself healthy in the pocketbook, you will be healthier everywhere.

17. **Rest.** This is essential to your health and I will give it its own chapter later.

18. **Don't Fear.** The Bible says;

"For God hath not given us the spirit of fear; but of power, and of love, and of a sound mind." 2 Timothy 1:7.

Unsound minds and fear come from Satan. I know we all face "down" times sometimes. I have had my share. But depression has a cause. Fix the cause and you fix the depression.

If you are depressed because you have lousy relationships, fix them. If you are depressed because you don't like what God has done or wants you to do, practice submitting. I know that it is a lot harder than it sounds, but with prayer, God can help you.

If you are depressed because you are mourning (someone close to you has died, you have lost a job, etc.) accept that depression is a normal part of the grief process. It is normal to be down. It hurts. My Hubby, who lost his parents in a car accedent when he was a teenager, told me after the loss of my mom, "It will always hurt. You just get used to the pain." Do you know, this really helped me. I quit feeling bad that I was still hurting, still depressed months later. It was normal. And he was right; several years have passed now, and I still hurt in a bitter-sweet way when I think of her, but it's not an overwhelming part of my day to day life now, I am no longer depressed. This is the normal process of time.

Sometimes the chemicals in the brain do malfunction and cause depression for no "life" reasons. If you can't finish the statement "I'm depressed because…" you may be looking at a chemical cause. Don't rule out things like blood sugar imbalance, allergens, or other envronmental causes. Do some reasearch. I do believe anti-depressents have their place in our world, but they are dangerous, personality changing drugs and should be your last result. Even then, give a try to St John's Wort (if you don't have heart disease) first. SJW has fewer side affects then perscription anti-depressents.

One big strategy to help pull yourself out of the "pit of despare" is to determine to show love and do to others what you wish they would do to you, not what they DO do to you. Quit focusing on how bad you feel and how others treat you and your relationships will change. Read your Bible and spend time praying so God can guide you into the place He wants you.

Remember step one to mental health? There is a God. If there is a God, He is in control. If God is in control and you are in the right place with Him, there is nothing to be afraid of. You are in God's hand.

19.   **Don't Naval Gaze.** A good deal of depression in our nation is caused by simple self-centeredness. The more you think about your problems the worse they get. Do something to make someone else feel better and you will feel better too. This is why the Bible tells us:

"Let nothing be done through strife or empty praise, but in humblness of mind let each esteem others better than themselves. Every one of you don't look out for just your own interests, but also for the interests of others. Let this mind be in you, which Christ Jesus also had." Philippians 2:5

God was giving us the path to mental health. Take care of others and your depression and mental illness will leave.

There is a good chance that if you do these things I have listed here, most if not all of your health problems will disappear. You need to care for your mental health first and foremost.

3. Life on the Farm

A Place to Start

I have always wanted to be a farmer and find it natural to refer to things in a "farm" setting. Since most humans were farmers throughout history, (until the 20th century), this is the way the vast majority of humans have lived. I think we will build us a mental farm to aid the discussion of nutrition. After all, all of our food still comes from a farm of some sort to begin with.

I picture a piece of property with a big white farm house in the middle of it. In the back to the left is a big red barn. Behind that are pastures and fields of grain. To the left of the house is a vegetable garden and in front of that an orchard. To the right and in front of the house is a small pond surrounded by nut trees with ducks and geese swimming in it. Directly in front of the house are a small herb garden and a big lawn filled with Dandelions and Plantain plants. Our farm has a small stream running through the pasture into the pond. Very picturesque and a refreshing place to swim in the summer. Hmm. I think it will snow here sometimes. Maybe we could learn to ice skate on our pond.

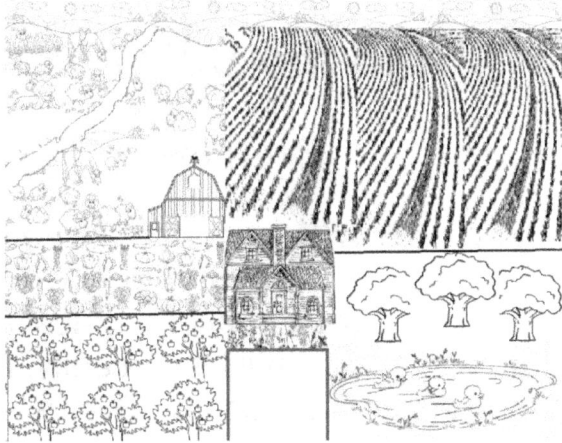

A food is "natural" if it could be grown on this ideal farm. It is unnatural if you need a factory and a bunch of petroleum to make it, and you could not possibly grow it yourself.

4. And the Spirit Moved

Exercise

"...let us run with patience the race that is set before us," Hebrew 12:1b

A farm takes a great deal of physical work to maintain. Farmers have, until just recently, been some of the healthiest members of society. They exercise daily as a matter of survival.

I have come to the conclusion that most Americans do not exercise nearly enough. For example, some estimates say those in third-world nations walk at least ten miles per day and Europeans walk five or more miles per day. Americans walk one-tenth of a mile! The three biggest causes of disease and general lack of health in America today are insufficient exercise, insufficient fiber, and insufficient water.

Exercise not only speeds up your metabolism (making your blood pump faster, allowing your organs to filter out toxins faster and better), it helps your digestion, works your heart, increases your insulin production and absorption, and balances your hormones.

I can hear the groans now. Everyone is having pictures of Workout videos, sweaty gyms, and old jogging shoes. That is not what I am talking about.

Our ancestors (the farmers) did not have these things, yet they did not have chronic heart disease, epidemic rates of Diabetes, or many other "modern ailments." The only ones who did the level of training we think we need to do in our culture were those training for the Olympics, or gladiator fights; the extreme warrior part of society. Truth is, this kind of training is very hard on your body and not really good for you in the long run.

The lower average maximum age of our ancestors can be mostly attributed to childhood diseases, bad sanitation, and lack of Penicillin. Today's modern plumbing coupled with antibiotics has assured that most of our children live until adulthood. A hundred years ago and in many third world countries today the infant mortality rate (babies dying before their fifth birthday) was/is around fifty percent. Imagine that; Half of your children dying before they could read! Oh, we are soooo blessed! Not only are odds good most of us will never know the pain of losing a child, we have enough food on our tables to make us worry about obesity. God is so good!

What I mean when I say "exercise" is simply increasing our physical activity. Imagine for a moment the workout our ancestors got just doing the laundry: haul the water (weight lifting), scrub the clothes on a wash board (underarm toner), wring the water out (arm, shoulder, wrist and hand strengthener), hang the clothes on the line (arm, shoulder, tummy, back workout), take the clothes down and iron them (more of the same). Today? Well we still have to carry the laundry to and from the machines but that is about it.

And think about baking bread (without the machine to do the kneading, ladies), washing dishes (not only without a machine, but haul your own water, too), washing soot covered walls (wood stoves were the only heat), ect.

Now, I am not about to give up my electronic servants in the name of exercise! I like Dianna

Dishwasher, Wanda Washing machine and Minnie Microwave. I am going to keep them around. But I think we can add some extra activity into the rest of our lives while building muscles and relieving stress.

You have probably read that we all need an hour a day of exercise. This is very true and being a perfectionist, when I decide to start exercising I sit down and design the "perfect" program that will work every muscle of my body, including my heart. I may spend three days doing this! Of course, I don't have the time or energy to actually do the exercises and if I try I am so sore the next day I can't move. Kind of defeats the whole purpose.

Instead, in the name of being a mere imperfect human, I am trying to add just a few things here and there, work it into my daily schedule like my ancestors did.

Walking is the best exercise, considering ease, cost, and the benefit to your body.

The first thing that comes to my mind is to park farther away from the store when I go shopping. That little extra walk can add up over time.

I try to make it a point to walk everyday (I'm not very good at it, but I try). Outside is best. The human body needs the sunshine remember. God designed us that way. The chemicals that cause depression decrease with exposure to the sun (and The Son, by the way). So whenever weather permits I go outside and take a walk, taking deep breaths, looking up and around at my surroundings, thanking God for the mountains, clouds, or whatever comes to mind.

How long of a walk should you take? Well, if you have not been walking much recently or are handicapped a three minute stroll away from your home is a good start. Just walk for three minutes then turn around and go back. Don't measure the distance. It doesn't matter. Everyday, walk a little bit longer (even just a minute or two). Don't push yourself too hard or you will burn out. Eventually you want to work up to 30-60 minutes each day.

If you can't walk outside, then walk inside. Around and around the coffee table. Your family will think you have flipped. You could put on good music and march! Kids would love it! Five whole minute's worth to start. Work your way up to more.

Put on some "kicking" music and dance your way through your housework (I like Carmen's "God's Got an Army").

You can buy a video to dance with or build a youtube.com favorites list once you are moving more. Have fun and enjoy.

Take the long way when you need to carry something to the other side of the house. Lift the same can up to the shelf and back down then up again when you put up groceries. Jump up and yell "Hallelujah!" throwing your arms in the air every time a commercial comes on TV. The inmates at the nuthouse your family puts you in will love it!

If you can't walk at all (and even if you can) do some weight lifting ("weight lifting" by the way, means "Pick up something heavy"). No, don't go spend hundreds of dollars on fancy iron weights. God gave you built in weights attached to your own body. Look at that thigh your knee is attached to. On even the skinniest person that is one heavy hunk of muscle! Stick your leg straight out and slowly lift your foot as high up off the ground as you can (you can do this sitting or standing). Then slowly lower it. If you can only do it once on each leg today, that is ok. That is more than you did yesterday! It works your thighs, tummy, back, hips and bottom. When you can do twenty or thirty lifts with ease, you can put heavy walking shoes on. When that is too easy, buy ankle weights (Wal-mart) or fill socks with sand and wrap them around your ankles and up the weight more. If you can do this standing then you can also lift your leg as far back as possible (with it straight) and as far to the side as possible. You can lift your arms up in the air the same way; stick them out in front of you and raise them up then lower them slowly. Stick them out to the sides and lift. That will work your shoulders, back, and chest muscles. Add cans of food or heavy books when your own arms are too easy. Dumbbells at Wal-Mart don't cost that much, either.

The more you lift weights, the stronger your muscles will get AND the more calories your body will burn when you are "couch potato-ing." That's right; it will raise your overall metabolic rate. Remember, that is like lowering your "miles per gallon," a good thing in people though a bad thing in cars.

You will want to work up to ten lifts, three or four times per day, but this may take awhile. Start slow.

Wal-mart also carries exercise bands. These are long plastic/rubber tubes with handles. They provide the same resistance training as weights for a fraction of the cost. You can hook them over a door or around a bed post. They often come with sample exercises or you can Google them.

4. And the Spirit Moved

While washing dishes, stand up on your toes. Up, down, up, down. Two times may be enough at first. Work up to twenty. Turn your toes in and repeat. Then point them out. Your whole body becomes the weight for your calves to lift.

When you sit up in bed, concentrate on using your tummy muscles to do as much of the lifting as possible.

Stretching your muscles helps them to not be as easily injured and makes them look leaner (and feels good). When you stand up, stretch up to the ceiling, and, if health permits, down to the floor. A couple times per day reach your hand over the top of your head and try to touch the wall on the opposite side. When you dry your foot after a shower, rest it on the highest surface you can (I can put mine on the bathroom counter) and streeetttchhh the hamstring muscles.

When you are walking, hold your tummy in (I have heard that this is actually the best tummy toner around) and squeeze your pelvic muscles. Stand up straight as much as you can; head up, shoulders down and back, back straight, tummy in, hips forward, toes straight ahead. You will look better (more alert, neater, smarter, nicer) immediately and will be strengthening the muscles to hold you that way, also preventing injuries.

If you are going to buy equipment to work out on, get a rebounder (miniature trampoline). Rebounding for ten minutes per day works every muscle group and increases circulation. Besides, it is fun!

You need to look around for some sort of fun activity. Now, some find those workout videos fit the bill. Most of us however don't. Consider joining a softball team, taking up horseback riding, going skating every

Caring for Your Masterpiece   43   MrsBettyTracy.com

Friday, planting a garden, buying a push lawn-mower, getting a dog, something active and fun. The funner it is the more likely you will do it.

If you have a smart phone, you can download a pedometer app and keep track of what you do each day. Set your goal number of steps to something low- maybe 3000- to start with. When you achieve this most days, raise the goal. You are ultimatly aiming for 10,000 steps per day on average.

It is also important to get up and move around each hour, especially if you have a desk job. We just aren't designed to sit still for long periods of time.

None of these things take very much. Any of them might be more then you are doing now. Every little bit helps. As you get healthier, you will feel stronger and want to do more. Be careful! You don't want to overdo it. You are in a marathon, not a sprint. **"Line upon line, precept upon precept, here a little there a little."** Isaiah 28:13. If you are unhealthy, it is most likely you didn't get into the condition you are in overnight. It took a long time. It will also take a long time to undo the damage and build your strength. And we must face it; we are older than we used to be. We will never be as healthy in our thirties or older as in our teens and twenties, but we can be better than we are now.

There are some health conditions that won't go away no matter what. Now don't get discouraged. I think we can all be healthier than we are right now, but some damage cannot be undone. We can have faith, though, that God will give us the strength to do what He has called us to do. He does not tell us to do things without giving us the ability to do them. If He has called you to a work that requires you to be healthier, then He will give you the strength and wisdom to get there. You just have to actually do it. Of course it works the other way around too; The stronger we are the more He can call us to.

At first, especially, you will be a little sore. If the pain is more than that, then cut back. You are overdoing it. If it is just annoying soreness, then keep on. It is your body saying "what are you doing to me? I don't want to work!" It will get used to it. Wait until the soreness goes away before you increase activity.

You don't have to do everything I have suggested; just one or two things is a good start. Or invent your own ways to up your activities and work your muscles (One woman I read about recently got rid of her dryer and set her basket of clothes on the ground to hang them on the line. She does purposeful deep knee bends while hanging the clothes up and taking them down. One day she counted and from washer to closet she did 500 deep knee bends!). It doesn't matter what you do, so use your imagination. Something is better than nothing!

Let's all **"present our bodies a living sacrifice unto God, holy, acceptable which is our reasonable** (not unreasonable) **service."** Romans 12:1

You are **"not your own. You are bought with a price."** 1 Corinthians 6:19, 20

That wonderful body you have belongs to Jesus. He bought it with His own blood. When you asked Him into your heart you gave yourself, including your body, to Him. He wants you to be wise in your use and care of it. And, yes, this means we must exercise.

Summary of Exercise:

- Stretch (reach and stretch and stand up straight)
- Move around (work up to about an hour a day, minimum). Also make sure you get up and move around at least once per hour.
- Pick up something heavy. (If lifting weights, start with your own body, work up to ten repetitions or lifts, ten times a day.)

5. Rest in the Lord

Rest and Sleep

"This is the rest wherewith you may cause the weary to rest; and this is the refreshing."
Isaiah 28:12

Our bodies need rest. This is a known fact of science. The question is, how much rest?

God made the night and day. I believe He intends for us to sleep every night and work in the day time. I understand that some people have jobs where they must work at night, but studies have shown that these people need an average of two more hours of sleep per day to make up for this unnatural pattern. And they tend to weigh more and suffer from more depression.

We should all get between six and ten hours of sleep per night. The older we get, the less sleep we generally need, so a child should have at least ten hours (babies may sleep for up to twenty at first) and an elderly person may only need six. Most of us should aim for eight. This allows our bodies to recuperate from the day's events.

Sleep deprivation can interfere with memory, energy levels, mental abilities, emotional mood (causing pessimism, sadness, stress and anger), exhaustion, fatigue and lack of physical energy, increase aging, and lowers our immune cells by 10-35%. It can drastically affect the body's ability to metabolize glucose (by as much as 40%), leading to symptoms that mimic early-stage Diabetes. Insufficient rest adversely affects the brain's ability to control speech, access memory, and solve problems. These physical reactions disappear when the person is allowed to rest properly.

Researchers have found that people who drive after being awake for 17 to 19 hours performed worse than those with a blood alcohol level of .05 percent. That's the legal limit for drunk driving in most western European countries. 16 to 60 percent of road accidents involve sleep deprivation. Road rage may be caused, in part, by a national epidemic of sleepiness.

"National epidemic of sleepiness?" Yes. We get an average of two hours less sleep per night than our "Dawn to Dusk" farmer ancestors did. Why? Electric lights, TV, cars that comfortably take us here and there, the 24/7 internet, etc. We are simply too busy and too involved to bother sleeping. Think about how different your life would be without electricity. When the sun goes down you light a fire in the fireplace and/or oil lamp. Then what? Read, talk to your family, play games, do hand crafts (This was a major time for education during the pioneer and colonial days). Still, you will be ready for bed before too long. Today the sun goes down and we flip a switch and continue working or watching the boob-tube into the wee hours of the morning. Then the alarm clock rings and we are up and at'em again.

First rule of rest: Sleep at night (10:00pm to 6:00am are the best times) at least eight hours. If you can't sleep, at least lie down and rest your body. Turn off the TV and computer and let your mind wander. If you have to do something, read a physical book.

You also need a weekly rest.

"And on the seventh day God ended his work which He had made, and He rested on the seventh

day from all his work which he had made." Genesis 2:2.

God worked for six days creating the world. Then He rested. Now this means, in part, that He simply quit creating on the seventh day. But it has more meaning;

"But the seventh day (of the week) **is the Sabbath of the LORD thy God. In it thou must not do any work, thou, nor thy son, nor thy daughter, thy manservant, nor thy maidservant, nor thy cattle, nor thy stranger that is within thy gates: because in six days the LORD made heaven and earth, the sea, and all that in them is, and rested the seventh day. That is why the LORD blessed the Sabbath day, and hallowed it."** Exodus 20:10

You see, because He had rested on the Sabbath, God told Israel to rest on the Sabbath. God wanted them to take one day per week to focus on Him and not work. Even their slaves and animals were not allowed to do any work. If Israel had followed this, what would have been the result? Their bodies would have had all the rest they needed to recuperate from the week's labor and they would have stayed home and spent time with their families and neighbors (you couldn't go very far without making your horse work). This would have been a mini vacation every week. Imagine how nice that would be?

Well, I don't have to imagine it. Though we are not "Sabbath keepers" in the traditional sense, we do consciously limit our Work and activities on Saturday night and Sunday. We have a simple meal and watch movies on Saturday night, spend the next morning fellowshipping and worshipping our God with or church family. We enjoy a good meal together and then go home and take a nap. That is followed by time being a family and enjoying family videos together with another simple meal. No chores, no cleaning, no school. Just rest and fun. A day to look forward to the whole week long. I really don't believe it matters if we take Sunday or Saturday or Tuesday off, but I think we should all take one day a week to focus on God and the wonderful gifts He has given us in our family and church family. This is a special time.

Not only does keeping a Sabbath make you rest your body and mind, it forces you to build a relationship with your family, preventing work-aholicism.

Have you ever wondered why we "need" vacations now but our ancestors didn't? Simple. The farmer got a vacation from pruning his orchard when it was time to plow the field. He got a vacation from plowing when it was time to plant and from planting when his animals started birthing. Then the sheep needed shearing, the berries picking and the garden planting. That was followed by haying, harvesting the fields then harvesting the garden. He vacationed from harvesting by shoring up the property for the winter and vacationed from that by sleeping until the late winter sun came up, doing inside repairs and chores, teaching his children to read and their other book work, and going to bed when the early winter sun went down. That would get tiring pretty fast so it is a good thing it only lasted a couple of months before he went on pruning vacation again.

This is why you need to take two weeks, minimum, per year off of your-same-ole- thing,-day-in-day-out-job (Most European countries require employers to provide six weeks of vacation). God made you to need at least some variety in your life. You need a rest from that schedule.

Rest rule three: Take a vacation every year (remember to turn your cell phone off!)

God also commanded Israel to have a special feast every New Moon. In other words, they were to be sure to have a party once per month. Imagine; some people think religion *stops* all the fun!

The new moon was to be celebrated with 1) blowing trumpets, 2) sacrifices, 3) worship in the house of God. Though Christians are not required to keep this feast, are even chided for doing so in Galatians, we need something to look forward to in our lives, even if it is as simple as taking one evening a month to get together with friends and visit. I think this is an important "rest" goal.

"Take my yoke upon you, and learn of me; for I am meek and lowly in heart: and you shall find rest for your souls." Matthew 11:29

Jesus is our rest. He provides us with spiritual rest, rest in our souls. Without Him we must worry and fret and figure out how to get everything done and what that even means. We must carry around the burden of sin and guilt on our shoulders. With Him we can just give it all away and He will throw the sins in the garbage, and tell us what needs to be done and what doesn't. He will guide us in how to go about doing what He wants us to do. We don't have to worry about it. In order to obtain this rest, we must first recognize that we are in need of His rest. We must first see that we are sinners.

"For all have sinned, and come short of the glory of God;" Romans 3:23.

"And so, since sin entered the world through one man, and death came by sin, and so death passed on to all humens, because all have sinned:" Romans 5:12.

There is not a human being that has ever walked this earth that has not sinned except Jesus Himself.

"For the wages of sin is death, but the gift of God is eternal life through Jesus Christ our Lord." Romans 6:23.

The tip-tiniest white lie deserves to be punished with eternal death; but Jesus paid that price for us. In order to receive His rest we must accept His gift of that payment. We must give Him our lives, our whole lives. Then we must seek Him.

Just like you spend time with your mate to build a relationship with him and to keep that relationship strong, you must spend time with Jesus.

Read your Bible everyday. This teaches you who He is, what He loves and what He hates.

Pray regularly. This keeps communication lines open so you can rest in His attention to you.

Yield your will to Him. Much like an escalator doesn't save you any work if you turn it off and climb the steps yourself, you must give God your all to get that rest in Him. Let Him handle it and don't worry anymore.

Summary: for sufficient rest...

- Sleep eight hours per night (more for children and if you are pregnant or ill.)

5. Rest in the Lord

- Take a "mini vacation" once per week; a day to not do any work or normal stuff, just worship, fellowship and fun.
- Make a point of doing something special once per month.
- Take at least two week's vacation per year.
- Take a daily rest with Jesus; read your Bible, pray and listen to Him giving Him all your burdens.

6. If Any Man Thirst

Water and What to Drink

"If any man thirst, let him come unto me, and drink."
John 7:37b

A very important way to care for the gift of our body that God has given us is to make sure we get enough water. God designed us to drink water, not sodas, sports drinks, or any other of our common beverages.

Water is the major component in our cells, including blood cells. I think about the Original Star Trek episode where the crew met a monster that removed the water from humans. All that would be left after an encounter with this creature was about two pounds of salt-like chemicals. This is not too very far from the truth. 65% of our body is water. Without water our body would literally starve to death. There would be no way for food to get to our cells to feed them.

Did you know that next to oxygen, water is the most essential nutrient for us to have? You can live about thirty days (give or take) without food, about three days without water, and about five minutes without air (without brain damage).

Most Americans don't get enough water (an estimated 75% are chronically dehydrated). We walk around suffering the effects of this dehydration; tiredness, edginess, slightly headachy, low endurance, fatigue (Lack of water is the #1 trigger of daytime fatigue), increased heart rate, impatience, difficulty in concentrating, dizziness, memory loss, and mental confusion. You know, in the country with the cleanest supply of water in the world it is strange that we don't drink enough.

Well, maybe not. We live in the culture of the skinny and chronically entertained. Anything to loose weight or have fun is considered ok (even if you don't need to loose weight). So, many women have taken pills to make them pee just so they can get into a smaller dress size. They drink as little (or NO!) water as possible to keep the pounds off. But look at the cost; Basic functioning is reduced. Quality of life goes down. And you know what? It's not real weight loss. They haven't lost a single ounce of fat. In fact, dehydration may cause your body to rely on carbohydrate fuel more than fat fuel, and it slows your metabolism by 3% short circuiting real weight loss!

And, of course, if it isn't a pretty color and doesn't tickle our "play" center we Americans won't drink it anyway.

Research says that 64-80 ounces (8 – 10 glasses or one big sports cup) of water a day is capable of significantly easing back and joint pain for up to 80% of people with those problems. Water lubricates your joints so you don't have bone grating on bone.

Drinking 5 glasses of water daily decreases the risk of constipation, and colon cancer by 45%, plus it is capable of slashing the risk of breast cancer by 79%, and you are 50% less likely to develop bladder cancer. This is because the water flushes the toxins that cause cancer out of your system.

Did you know that **we absorb as much water through our skin when we shower** as when we drink? So not only is it important to bathe regularly to wash off germs, look and smell better, but we need it to help keep ourselves hydrated. It is best to install a whole house filter if you can so you are drinking and bathing in the purest water possible. City water is treated with chlorine, which is better than bathing in germs, but still not really good for you.

Drink before you are thirsty. If you wait until you get thirsty you have waited too long. I find that if I keep a bottle of water by me at all times, I will sip on it throughout the day and not even realize it. This is the best way I have found for me to keep hydrated. For some people, it helps to add a squirt of lemon juice to their water or make sure they have plenty of ice. In fact, the colder the water you drink the more it raises your basic metabolism. It takes more energy to warm up cold water to body temperature then tepid water.

Additional benefit: Water is free. Unlike a daily 20-ounce bottle of soda that will cost you $10.00 a week, tap water costs you nothing. That's $520.00 in savings per year!

Other Drinks

Soda
What else should we drink? Most people in our sociezty drink sodas almost exclusively. This is not a good idea. Other than entertainment, there is no redeeming value to sodas. For starters, Caffeine increases the excretion of calcium, increasing the risk of osteoporosis, (Female athletes that drink sodas have significantly more bone breaks than those that don't.)

The Artificial colorings in most sodas have been linked to ADHD as well as certain allergies.

The carbonation eats the enamel off your teeth.

The other chemicals cause kidney stones, increase the risk of heart disease and act like a diuretic (making you pee more, thus be more dehydrated, function less efficiently, feel more hungry, and more thirsty causing you to drink more soda which makes you pee more which...) and increase the risk of obesity (you take in sweet, whether real or artificial, and your body says "Hey! I need vitamins to digest this sweet!" So you grab a Twinkie because your brain interprets the vitamin craving as a sugar craving. Your body screams for more vitamins, you give it more sugar, and so on). In fact, the single biggest source of calories in most American's diet is soda (as much as a full fourth of their daily calorie intake).

Imagine eating seven to nine teaspoons of sugar straight. That's how much sugar is in a twelve-ounce can of soda; and we drink the stuff by the gallon! Many people have lost weight by simply eliminating soda entirely from their diet.

And on the effectiveness of diet sodas; have you ever seen a skinny person drinking one? Could the extra sweet of our artificial sweeteners increase our cravings for food making our overall intake of calories go up? There is increasing evidence that this is what is happening. (More about artificial sweeteners later, but remember that the chemical composition of Nutri Sweet is the same as formaldehyde).

There are no vitamins in soda and very few minerals, most of which we all get plenty of anyway (such as salt).

No, stay away from sodas as much as possible. Occasionally it's ok (I usually have one or two per week).

Our bodies can handle some unnecessary junk, but they should be a rare treat. The less the better.

Coffee

Coffee's value is still up to debate. It appears that caffeine prevents the formation of kidney stones, while it is leaching the calcium from our bones. Coffee itself appears to lower the risk of Parkinson's disease, Diabetes, tooth decay, Alzheimer, and cancer. But it can also badly affect the heart if you are already having trouble. Coffee has over 1000 different chemicals, half of which are known carcinogens. However, carrots also have chemicals that, by themselves, are carcinogens. Take any such statistics with a grain of salt.

Caffeine is a natural "pesticide" given off by the bean to keep the bugs from eating it. A cup of coffee contains about 120 mg of caffeine. If you injected that amount of caffeine directly into your blood, you would die. The rush of energy you get from your coffee is your body speeding up your metabolism to get rid of this insecticide. Your body takes water from everywhere to help flush the stuff out. Of course, a speeding metabolism (more than 100 calories a day's worth) helps you lose weight if you need to, so coffee drinkers have an easier time with weight control.

I began drinking coffee a couple of years ago, mostly for help with my migraines (coffee causes the blood vessels in the head to dialate, releaving or preventing many headaches.) I have benefitted some from the side affect of more ability to consentrate, sence coffee helps stimulate the "self-control" nerves in the brain, making it great for those with Attention Defecit Disorder.

Whether coffee is over all good for you, or bad, it certainly is better for you than soda.

If you do decide to drink coffee, limit those pre-made coffee drinks sold in grocery stores. They are generally made with LOTS of added sugar and bad fats destroying any benefits from the coffee itself. Those Yuppie coffee shops aren't generally much if any better (and in a blind taste test the much cheaper McDonalds beat them out anyway.)

Kool-Aid
When you sit down with a glass of Kool-Aid the main ingredient is water (good). The second is sugar (bad). Then you will find artificial flavorings and preservatives (petroleum products) as well as some natural preservatives (citric acid, otherwise known as vitamin C.) All in all, it is healthier to drink Kool-Aid than soda, BY FAR, but water or juice would be better.

Lemon Ade
If you make it yourself, (lemon juice with sugar or honey to sweeten it) down right good for you. If you buy it pre-made it will have some preservatives and possibly artificial flavorings and colorings. That has to weigh in. I don't think God wanted us to eat petroleum and most preservatives are actually poisons if taken alone (that is why they work. They kill the bugs that cause food to spoil). Avoid them when possible. But once again, lemon ade beats soda hands down.

Bottled Water
There really isn't an advantage to bottled water over tap unless you just like the flavor enough that it makes you drink more. In fact, if you are on city water, it is very

likely that what comes out of your tape has met far more stringent government regulation for cleanliness than what is in the bottle. Bottled water simply isn't that regulated, though many companies just fill their bottles with whatever comes out of their tap. Those waters would meet the fed's standards.

Vitamin Water

Many manufacturers have discovered that if they add a bunch of vitamins and herbs to water people will pay more money. Unfortunately, most of them also add a bunch of cheap sugars to make you like their product better. Most of the time, the number of calories in these products far outweighs any benefit from the vitamins and herbs. You would be better off taking a multi vitamin and drinking plain 'ole H_2O.

By the way, the same goes for energy drinks.

Flavored water

Again, read the ingredients. Water, good. Sugar, bad. "Diet" water? Sweetened with chemicals that do not occur in God's nature; we can't grow them on our farm. Same for the flavorings; more petro-chemicals. Now, home made fruit water made with pure water with a dash of fruit juice added is good for you. Enjoy!

Sports drinks

God did not create a Sport's Drink Tree for a reason. Generally speaking, water will do everything you need without the calories and chemicals in sports drinks. The only exception is for those that engage in long, strenuous activity, such as Olympic sports or hard physical labor (those, like my hubby, who work in warehouses- pseudo-ovens- all day in summer may fit this category also). These people lose enough minerals that they do need the artificial replacement of sports drinks, though some recent studies say chocolate milk works even better. The decision to drink them should be balanced with the knowledge of the number of calories and chemicals you are getting also. They are very high in sugar and salt.

Juices

Watch this one carefully. Most "juices" on the store shelves have added sugar (watch out for the words "drink," and "cocktail." They signal extreme amounts of sugar have been added). Totally unnecessary. Those that are labeled 100% fruit juice should still be diluted 50/50 with water. The straight juice lost a good deal of its water during processing.

You will get the vitamins from the fruits and veggies in their juices, but you won't get the fiber that eating the real thing would give you. Actually, I consider milk and juice to be foods, not drinks. They are full of food-like nutrition. Juice you could do fine without, but it is a nice treat, especially if you are trying to wean away from sodas. Try mixing different flavors to make them even more interesting.

Tea

Tea is a fascinating subject. Tea is the water that is left after you pour it (boiling or very hot) onto plant leaves and let it sit for a few minutes. The health benefit of tea varies depending on what kind of leaves you use.

What most people think of as "tea" is from the Camellia plant. It has a few vitamins and minerals and has been shown to have some benefit to the human body, such as possibly preventing cancer, tooth decay, diabetes, heart disease, wrinkles, hypertension and obesity. (This is another drink I never really learned to like). The caffeine, though, is not good for you (see Soda and Coffee).

Caffeine could be considered a natural upper, but I, personally, don't think it is good to give yourself an "up" off of chemicals no matter how natural. If you are depressed, find out the cause and fix it. If you are tired, take a nap or go to bed earlier (though occasional circumstances may necessitate the use of caffeine as an upper. As long as it isn't a regular means of functioning it won't hurt you). As I have said, Americans tend to be sleep deprived as much as they are dehydrated. We compensate for it by drinking drugs to keep us going. Keeping yourself going by using chemicals will wear your body out faster; make your brain not function right, and cause major health problems down the road. It is much better to listen to your body and do what it is telling you it needs. If you are tired, then sleep. If you are thirsty, then get a glass of water and drink it.

Black tea (which boosts the immune system and heart function) is what you get when you ferment, oxidize and cook the Camellia leaves. (This is "normal" tea tea)

Green tea (which helps hypertension, and possibly bone health) is unprocessed.

Herbal teas are teas made from any other plant.

Black and Green tea contain caffeine. Studies have shown that tea helps to burn fat faster. They don't yet know if it is a chemical reaction to caffeine combined with the catechin found in tea or just the catechin alone. I also discovered that the drinking of green tea has been linked to higher rates of anti-oxidants (cancer fighters). Black tea (Lipton, instant teas, etc.) have some of the same benefits, but not in nearly the same amounts. Again, choose tea over soda any day, as long as it isn't those pre-made, over-fatted, over sugared types in the store. Read the labels. A (very) few of the premade teas are actually just tea with a hint of sugar but most have way too much junk.

I have recently tried peppermint tea for the first time. This is made from peppermint leaves. That's it. It is very refreshing and aids digestion by calming the stomach and toning the muscles of the digestive tract. Have mild indigestion or just want a refreshing after dinner drink? Try peppermint tea.

Raspberry leaf tea (yes, that is the complete ingredient list) is a time honored (and pleasant) drink for women to use to strengthen their reproductive tracts. It can be taken at any time of life (puberty through menopause, pregnant, nursing, in between, etc.) and I have seen recommendations for doses from one to three cups per day. It will also pleasantly relieve upset tummies in children and men as well as provide many vitamins and minerals; enough to classify raspberry leaves as a food instead of a medicinal herb.

Chamomile tea is a time honored nerve relaxant.

Clove tea will help you sleep.

Honey/Lemon tea (approximately 1 Tablespoon each to one cup of water and heat. Adjust for flavor) will sooth a sore throat. I could go on.

My advice would be to research thoroughly any tea you want to drink and make sure you are willing to risk any side effects (All medicines have side effects, even natural ones. The naturals just tend to have fewer, less sever ones than the over the counter or prescription ones.)

As far as regular tea, again do some research and see if the benefits (many) out weigh the detriments (some) to you. The answer to this will be different for different people.

Alcohol

"Wine is a mocker and beer a brawler; whoever is led astray by them is not wise." Proverbs 20:1

"He who loves pleasure will become poor; whoever loves wine and oil will never be rich." Proverbs 21:17

"Do not join those who drink too much wine or gorge themselves on meat, for drunkards and gluttons become poor, and drowsiness clothes them in rags." Proverbs 23:20, 21

"Who has woe? Who has sorrow? Who has strife? Who has complaints? Who has needless bruises? Who has bloodshot eyes? Those who linger over wine, who go to sample bowls of mixed wine. Do not gaze at wine when it is red, when it sparkles in the cup, when it goes down smoothly! In the end it bites like a snake and poisons like a viper. Your eyes will see strange sights and your mind imagine confusing things. You will be like one sleeping on the high seas, lying on top of the rigging." Proverbs 23:29-34

"It is not for kings, O Lemuel, not for kings to drink wine, not for rulers to crave beer, lest they drink and forget what the law decrees, and deprive all the oppressed of their rights. Give beer to those who are perishing, wine to those who are in anguish; let them drink and forget their poverty and remember their misery no more." Proverbs 31:4-7

"Drink no longer water, but use a little wine for thy stomach's sake and thine often infirmities." 1 Timothy 5:23

(God made) "wine to make them glad, olive oil to soothe their skin, and bread to give them strength." Psalms 104:15

The claim is that alcohol consumed in moderate quantities (1-3 drinks per day. A drink is a twelve ounce can or bottle of beer, a five ounce glass of wine, or 1.5 ounces of liquor [either straight or in a mixed drink]) lowers your risk of many, many diseases. I question much of this. Solomon certainly didn't seem to think alcohol was usually a good thing, though the Bible as a whole is not dogmatic.

Many of the studies showing benefits were very poorly done, making them unreliable. Those who don't drink are often ex-alcoholics (who suffer from very poor health), or are abstaining because they are taking medicine for other conditions (not exactly a reliable "abstainer" group to compare health with). Alcoholics are often heavy smoking, non-exercising, non-religious (bad for your physical health), bad eating individuals, and many ex-drinkers only change the drinking part of their life style. Lumping ex-drinkers in with life long abstainers will certainly not give a clear enough picture of the helath of consuming or not consuming alcohol.

Many point out that the French have the highest consumption of alcohol per person and the second lowest rate of heart disease (after Japan). But there are many variables here. Among those countries studied, France has the highest per capita wine consumption (wine is relatively low in alcohol and high in vitamins), high vegetable consumption and moderate consumption of bad fats. In other words, the French eat so well the alcohol may not have anything to do with their lower rates of heart disease.

A recent study carefully distinguished between former drinkers and long-term abstainers. Using this distinction, the supposed health benefits for light drinkers over long-term abstainers were disproven for both men and women. When they factored out the ex-drunks, those that never drank at all were healthier than those that drank a little.

An unborn baby can easily be damaged by mommy drinking alcohol. Brain damage, facial disfigurement, growth retardation, and overall reduced brain size often occurs.

Serotonin (the anti- depression chemical produced by the brain) is a factor for brain development. Serotonin is significantly decreased in a fetus exposed to ethanol. Pregnant women should not drink alcohol.

The cancer rate in alcoholics is ten times higher than that in the general population. Studies find a much lower incidence of cancer among groups (such as

Mormons and Seventh-Day Adventists) who abstain from alcohol (though non-smoking, a religious life style, and faith in God are certainly factors, too).

Even one drink per day is associated with a 9% increase in breast cancer; four drinks with a 21% increased risk of prostate cancer. Nearly half of all cancers in the mouth and throat have been attributed to alcohol.

Too much alcohol can **suppress the immune system**, leading to increased susceptibility to infections.

Alcohol is addictive. You need more and more of it to get the same effect and need that "hit" more often. Alcohol withdrawal symptoms include tremors, anxiety, variations in body temperature and potentially fatal convulsions. Reread the verses from Proverbs above.

Alcohol has seven calories per gram. That is three more calories per gram than protein (milk) or carbohydrates (juice or even soda). There is a reason it is called a "beer belly."

There is a correlation between alcohol consumption and early death. **Accidents are the biggest cause of death before age sixty** and alcohol is the biggest cause of accidents (note: this is changing as Marujuana is begin legalized all over). Drunk driving is the biggest cause of car accident deaths, accounting for a full one third. And half of the car deaths in the 25-29 year age group are from alcohol. My hubby's own parents were killed by a 22 year old drunk driver.

32% of fatal falls, 42% of fatal fires/burns, 34% of fatal drownings, 29% of fatal poisonings, 32% of homicide victims and 23% of suicide victims are due to someone being drunk.

And intoxication is at least, if not entirely, the cause of more than half of all cases of **domestic violence.**

In other words, alcohol, at least in excess, makes you stupid.

Why did Paul, then, tell Timothy to "Take a little wine for thy stomach's sake?" My research says that the wine drunk during the time of the Roman Empire was the same as if you took today's wine and watered it down half and half with water, somewhere around the alcohol content of a wine cooler. So, for starters, they didn't get ethanol in the same amount. The naturally dehydrating part of alcohol is counteracted by the extra water, better flushing toxins from your system.

Secondly, they didn't have the modern water systems we have. Likely, Timothy was suffering from dysentery, a disease often carried by drinking-water. The alcohol in the low-alcohol wine they commonly drank would have killed the dysentery bacteria as well as other harmful bacteria. We add chlorine to our water for the same purpose. Not sure which one is better, to tell you the truth.

Why did Jesus make wine out of water at the wedding in Canaan? There are some benefits to wine. It is made of grape juice and is high in the same good antioxidants, vitamins and minerals that grape juice is high in (though a hand full of berries has even more of these same benefits). In small amounts, it does improve the mood in most people, thus increasing the enjoyment of such a celebration as a wedding. I don't think there is anything wrong with this (isn't it nice of me to not think Jesus did anything wrong?) An occasional drink for celebration purposes won't hurt anything.

The problem is that in this society, we rely on alcohol to help us feel good, to forget our problems and make us relax. We use it like a drug, not like a party favor.

Solomon said to give drink to those who are in great pain or dying. Do you fit that category? If you do, you need to do something to fix your pain. Physical pain can't always be cured in this life. I see no problem with using what you need to help you function. Take comfort that there is coming a day when you won't hurt anymore if you have Jesus in your heart. If you don't, ask Him into your heart now or, well, get used to the pain. It will only get worse.

God has a purpose for everything He created, including alcohol. It is good as a disinfectant, pain killer and the occasional party treat. But just like everything else, it can cause great damage when used wrongly. I don't use it at all (except as a disinfectant). When anything begins to smell like that in my refrigerator, I throw it away.

(Note on marujuna: MJ has many of the same problems as alcohol. It does very much have sid affects, but not really any more than drinking does. There are some health benefits, too. Much research is being done right now on the affects of MJ on cancer. There may be a cure luring in there somewhere.)

7. These are Weighty Matters

How Important is Weight

We all know there is an obesity epidemic in the US. Ahhh, actually, no, we don't know this.

Yes, the "average American" is more likely to be classified as obese now than they were 30-40 years ago, but that isn't an obesity epidemic.

<u>Some interesting facts:</u>

The government lowered the number that qualifies a person as "obese." Why? According to the panel responsible, they were under extreme pressure to align America's official standard with the World Health Organization's standard (note that they did not say they were bringing America in line with any research.)

Why did the WHO set their standard where they set it? Political pressure to align with the International Commission on Weight's standard.

Who is the ICW? A political action group funded by the two pharmaceutical companies that make the majority of weight loss medicines.

Does anyone else smell something fishy?

So one morning a large number of Americans who were "normal weight" when they went to bed woke up legally obese so that the drug companies could sell more weight loss medicines.

Minorities have always averaged a higher weight than whites in America. Over the last few decades, the white birth rate has fallen to such an extent that minorities are making up a bigger and bigger percentage of the population. This means that, though no one is necessarily any fatter, the "average" weight is higher.

If there is an actual average weight gain in America (and we aren't really sure yet), there are several possible causes:

We no longer have times of famine. This is a GOOD thing for overall health, even if we do have to wear a bigger size dress.

We have great house heaters. It takes less energy to keep warm in the winter, so we use less to stay alive than we used to, again, much better for overall health than nearly freezing to death every winter.

We don't really have any idea what vaccines do in the very long run. We do know that populations who are vaccinated have a way higher rate of type 2 Diabetes, obesity and cancer. Type 2 Diabetes is caused by our cells refusing to take in insulin. Why are American cells suddenly insulin resistant; and at about sixty years after mass vaccination took place, too? It is the taking in of insulin that allows us to burn calories[6]. Is it that the vaccinations themselves causing diabetes, or that the money that allows us to afford vaccinations also allows other habits that cause obesity and diabetes? We don't know yet.

The vast majority of babies in America have been fed **artificial breastmilk** (formula) for several decades now. It is a known fact that one (of many!) advantages of

---

[6] The most rescent research suggests that our cells quit taking in insulin BEFORE we gain the weight associated with Diabetes. It is the Diabetes that is causeing the weight gain, not obesity causing the Diabetes.

breastfeeding is lower obesity rates as adults. Babies simply don't get the right nutrition from formula to form healthy bodies.

Meat producers give their animals estrogen in order to make them gain weight faster.

Dairy farmers give their cows estrogen in order to make them produce more milk.(This is less and less true since consumer demand has caused many dairies to stop this practice).

Doctors give women estrogen in order to keep them from having babies (the major components of The Pill are estrogen and progesterone). These hormones are then peed into the water supply by the women, so men, especially in big cities get them too.

Pesticides, herbicides, and most household cleaners contain chemicals that our bodies interpret as estrogen.

Many processed foods contain soybeans which are very high in phyto-estrogens.

Now to repeat the first sentence in the last paragraph; Meat producers give their animals estrogen in order to make them gain weight faster. Can we all say a collective "Duhhhh"?

Meat producers also **feed their animals corn** to encourage weight gain.

Corn (especially in the form of corn syrup) is now in all of our food from our sodas to our spaghetti sauce to some kinds of potato chips. It is processed faster in the human body than other grains, not giving time for the body to use the calories before it has to do something with them. So the body stores them.

Also, recent studies say that a corn derivative, **High Fructose Corn syrup**, suppresses the production of the hormone that tells our brains we are full and don't need any more food. (This is not to say, "Don't eat corn." The whole grain is a nutritious food, quite good for us. It's the processed product that is causing problems).

Processing food removes fiber, B vitamins, chromium, iodine, magnesium and manganese. Fiber helps food move along and fills the tummy so you don't eat as much. The vitamins and minerals are responsible for helping us to use the calories we take in. Without these nutrients the calories just sit around (in the form of fat) waiting for something to come along and use them.

Dehydration and sleep deprivation can cause the metabolism to slow down and retain more weight. Americans are chronically dehydrated and sleep deprived.

We also exercise a good deal less. Since the invention of cars, computers and television, we have all become far more sedentary.

And don't forget those "labor saving" devices we all have in our homes. They should be called "exercise stoppers" instead. Just imagine how much more exercise you would get if cars and electricity were outlawed. With everything combined that is needed to produce, prepare, and clean up from our meals plus clothe our families, plus maintaining a basic cleanliness in our homes (no vacuum, remember. You have to sweep the floors.), we would get far more exercise and all the gyms in town would probably close.

Instead we all spend hours every day staring at a TV or computer and munching on empty calories.[7] The amazing thing really is that we don't have greater health problems than we do!

Add to all this that **our bodies were designed to store extra weight** to prepare for famine and when famine comes, our metabolism slows down, using fewer calories, in order to keep us alive until things get better. It does this by "eating" its own muscle. Since muscle takes more calories to stay alive than fat does, as the muscle disappears the body's calorie needs fall. A simple and necessary survival mechanism.

Unfortunately, our bodies don't know the difference between dieting and famine. When we quit dieting, we eat the same amount of calories we did before the diet, but now we have less muscle to keep alive. This is why we put on more weight after a diet than we lose during it.

Yes, you are not the only one who gains it all back. In fact, **less than 5%** of people who lose weight keep it off for five years or more. In one study, those who had lost weight began putting it back on after just six months even though they were eating **fewer** calories and exercising **more** than when they lost the weight. This is how powerful the mechanism God created to keep us from starving to death is! Our bodies will simply fight any weight loss with all their power. There really isn't much you can do about it no matter how hard you try, no matter how much you deny yourself.

This is sure a Doom and Gloom section!

---

[7] Empty Calorie= a calorie with few or no vitamins, minerals, or fiber. Something that causes a net loss of nutrients to the body.

Good News #1: Being fat doesn't mean you have a lack of self-control. Oh, once in a while you run into someone who really does eat enough for two or three people every day, but most of the time fat people don't eat any more than skinny people, sometimes not as much. In fact, those fat people I have known in my life are some of the most disciplined, health conscious, self-controlled people I have ever met. That's actually probably why they're fat; all the self-control applied to eating causes their bodies to continually be in famine mode, hoarding every possible calorie so they don't starve!

The fact is that you haven't failed at all! All the diets and programs you have tried have been flawed! They are what has failed! (Think about it; if any diet program actually worked, wouldn't we all be skinny? Wouldn't it be the only program left because it's what everyone flocked to?)

Diets and weight loss programs don't take into account that wonderful mechanism God has put in our bodies that keeps our weight at a steady point.

Good News #2: Being fat isn't as bad for you as we are led to believe.

First of all, we must always remember where the money comes from no matter the issue. TV shows, including news programs, survive by attracting advertisers. If they offend their advertisers, they go broke. Next time you watch TV count how many of the commercials are for the drug companies (who all make a fortune on weight loss medicines). No TV program is going to tell you it's ok to be "Pleasingly Plump" because they will lose a major income source if they do. Same goes for magazines. Any media really.

It seems that the markers for ill health (i.e. high blood pressure) only occur in those fat people who have dieted. Those in countries where obesity is a sign of wealth and intelligence don't have high blood pressure or any other ill-health markers, no matter how fat they are.

A better marker for health is performance on a treadmill. Fat men who could perform at a "fit" level had the same death rates as skinny men who performed as "fit," and LOWER death rates than skinny men who didn't do well on the test. It's the fitness level that matters, not the padding on the belly.

Why do studies say it's so unhealthy to be fat? It seems our studies just don't look at their evidence close enough.

It's poverty, not obesity, that is unhealthy. Poor people can't afford to live in healthier neighborhoods, buy organic (if any) fruit, join gyms and softball teams, and have many other factors[8] that cause them to be both heavier and unhealthier. It isn't their weight that is unhealthy. It is the poverty that causes both the weight and the ill health.

Heavier people can stand high blood pressure better than skinny people[9]. They have a much lower rate of both heart attack and stroke than skinnies with high

---

[8] If your child asks you for a bicycle, new coat, and a can of coke, and all you can afford is the coke, you will buy the coke, even if you know it is not really healthy for him. You simply can't afford anything else and it is bad for a child to always be told "no." Once in a while he genuinely needs a "yes."

[9] Of course, this could be because many doctors use too small blood pressure cuffs for fat people giving false high readings. In other words, fat people who read with high blood pressure with a skinny cuff often read perfectly normal with a big cuff.

blood pressure. In fact, as our average, national weight has risen, our rates of heart disease have fallen, occur later in life, and have become more survivable. Only part of this can be attributed to better treatment. Some is the protection of the extra weight.

Our goals should not be to get as skinny as possible. That's Holywood speaking.[10] The dieting necessary for that robs our bodies of nutrients it needs to prevent ill health.

Our goals should be to be as healthy as possible. This is not accomplished by obsessing over food and exercise. That is a sign of the mental illnesses that fall under "eating disorder." Think about it; if skinny people act like fat people about food or exercise, we say they are mentally ill and need help (anorexia and bulimia).

Our goals should be to be healthy. This means to eat right, exercise and have the right mental health.

A group of hotel maids had their health numbers measured. Then they were taught about the benefits of getting proper exercise. Half of them were then told how their everyday work met those exercise goals. This half saw significant improvement in their numbers within a couple of weeks without changing a thing they were doing. Just knowing they were already begin healthy, made them healthier. There's that placebo affect again.

I would advise you to NOT have the weight lose surgeries. Again, they have not been around long enough

---

[10] Since fat is an ancient sign of wealth (and Americans really do hate the rich) and in modern times a sign of poverty (which Americans also hate and pretend don't exist) our culture gets us coming and going with the result of simply hating anyone who is fat for the fat's sake.

for us to know the long term consequences twenty or thirty years down the road. There is a good chance they shorten your lifespan by reducing your absorption of necessary nutrients. We do know people die from these surgeries and that some get very ill. An alarmingly high number of people put the weight back on after a few years. This all defeats the goal of being healthier, what we are supposed to be having the surgury for in the first place!

Some hints on what our focus should really be:

Many times we eat when we are really thirsty, so drink lots of water. Buy an ice water, tea, coffee or lemon ade when you eat out instead of a soda, and keep a glass of water by you throughout your day if possible. (I have heard of people losing all their excess baggage by just quitting the soda habit. Since soda is not good for you under any circumstances, the weight is really irrelevant by itself. It's just a sign of a problem.)

Remember to slow down, taste your food, and enjoy the experience of eating. Play slow music. The beat will help you slow down. Not only are you less likely to choke, but you will absorb your food and nutrients much better. Also, the emotional satisfaction of eating will be there sooner if you chew slowly and pay attention to the texture and flavor of your food. God made food pleasing and we need to enjoy it. I don't know about anyone else, but I find myself gulping my food down without even tasting it (much like a vacuum cleaner!) then, later, I get the desire to eat something. Not hunger, mind you. An emotional need to put things in my mouth and chew. When I take small bites, taste the food and notice the texture I seldom have that case of "munchies" later on. Munchies are often fulfilled with foods that disrupt health. They make you sick. If, however, you munch on healthy foods (i.e. veggie sticks) eat away! Munch all you like.

This goes for eating in front of the TV also. Those who watch the boob-tube while eating their meals have been scientifically shown to absorb fewer vitamins and minerals. In fact, making it a rule that no one eats, not even just a cookie, without sitting at the table with a plate, makes it even more memorable every time you eat and makes it harder to eat what you shouldn't be eating anyway (and keeps the crumbs in the dinning room and kitchen making the house easier to clean to boot!)

DON'T SKIP BREAKFAST! Studies have shown that those who do not eat breakfast consume more calories per day than those that do. You will eat more for lunch and supper than you would have if you had eaten breakfast.

Even if you only have a cup of yogurt and a slice of toast, eat something. Supper to lunch is way too long for your brain to go without fuel. Eating breakfast keeps your metabolism from going into starvation mode and slowing down. In fact, many have better success with weight control when they eat every two or three hours. This keeps the metabolism functioning at peak speed and keeps your brain running on an even keel.

Research your favorite fast food restaurants on the internet. They all have websites that detail their nutrient content. It isn't automatically bad to eat out. It doesn't make a food less healthy because someone else prepares it. It matters what the food is and HOW it's made. Some restaurants are very unhealthy with nothing desent on the menu. But some are down-right good for you. For the type of things I eat, Wendy's can be even healthier than eating at home! They make their salads with a variety of fresh greens I don't keep around the house and their chili can only be matched at home by making it by scratch, something I don't have the time to do often. And Wendy's uses a high fiber potato for their baked potatoes and French fries to boot! Yes, you need to do the research for yourself and be an informed shopper. Few can avoid eating out altogether, so be prepared when you do to make wise choices.

Keep a journal of everything you put into your mouth. Now, I don't want you to count your calories. I want you to record what you eat and how you feel 15 and 30 minutes later. Do you feel tired or energetic? Happy or depressed? This will help you to know what foods react well to your body, and which ones are causing a problem. We aren't all made the same, and foods don't always do the same thing to each of us. Know what makes YOU feel best and stick to that.

When shopping, compare labels on everything. I like raisin bran for breakfast. But there are many different brands to choose from. By doing a little comparison I found out that:

- Kellogg's has 190 calories, 6.5 grams of fiber, and 5.1 grams of protein per cup.
- Post has 187 calories, 7.7 grams of fiber and 4.7 grams of protein.
- But Fiber One has 170 calories, 11 grams of fiber and 4 grams of protein.

So by choosing a different brand of the same food I am going to eat anyway I add 4.5 extra grams of fiber, a nutrient most Americans are seriously lacking in. This is enough fiber to hold off many digestive problems. And I discovered Fiber One tastes better to boot! (The lower protein doesn't matter since the milk I add has more than enough).

Avoid preservatives and flavorings (buy organic if possible). They are added to keep the food from spoiling and make them taste better (because factory processing destroys flavors), but have the nasty side effect of stimulating the part of the brain that increases hunger. This works well for the manufacturers because you then buy more food and they make a bigger profit. But the effect on you is not good.

What should you actually eat? Should you eat carbs and limit proteins? Avoid carbs and indulge in fats? Only eat at certain times per day or eat certain foods together?

I have taken all the major diets (Atkins, Food Combining, Low fat, Heart Smart, etc.) and compared them. They all have a few things in common;

- eat more fresh veggies, fresh fruits, whole grains,
- and (if you eat them) make your meats and dairy unprocessed (no cold cuts, lunch meats, American cheese, or "processed cheese foods" whatever that is;
- do grass fed and organic if possible. I don't because I simply can't afford it).
- Avoid white sugar, white flour, "bad fats," and things processed (don't even allow them in your house. Very few cases of chocolate cravings are powerful enough to make you get in your car and drive to the store. If it

isn't in your house, you probably won't eat it. And your kids get more than enough of them outside the house).
• Exercise more.

If you just do these things you actually obey 90% of all the requirements of all the different diet plans.

So, what do you eat?

Whatever you want (unprocessed breads, grains, fruits, veggies, meats, dairy, etc). A study observed a bunch of two year olds playing. They were given all types of good foods and allowed to go get whatever they wanted any time they wanted. The result was that over the course of an average week, each child ate a balanced diet by instinct. Oh, one might eat nothing but fruit for a couple of days, but then their natural appitites would have them eating meat for a day. It all averaged out. This confirms to me that God gave us an instinct for what we need if we can just ignore all the static of our culture trying to tell us otheriwse.

When you want it. Listen to your body. It will tell you when you need more.

Enjoy the variety of good foods God has made for us.

And exercise more.

I find the human body fascinating. God sure did a good job when He made it. Did you know that the human being is the only thing God called "Very Good" when He finished it? Everything else He just called "Good." God gave you your body as a special gift, a house to live in for your whole life. It is not automaticly broken just because it is bigger than the latest fashion model's body. It is your responsibility to take care of this house: do the maintenance, so to speak. He gave us everything we need to care for it.

Think about what Christ did on the cross for us. He took that special body He had and broke it to give us life. I believe the Bible teaches us that that life is physical as well as spiritual. We are living under the curse of Adam right now. That is why we get sick and hurt and eventually die. But our true selves are eternal. We can choose eternal death with no relief from pain and illness. Just constant dying. Or we can choose eternal life with Jesus. Never any more pain. Christ provided that choice for us when He chose to die on the cross. What do you choose? Life or death?

8. Eat healthier

Basic Philosophy

"And he made them a feast, and they did eat and drink." Genesis 26:30

We hear "eat healthier" every where, but what does it mean? There are many different opinions, but my research has found some guidelines that basically agree with them all, even the umpteen different government food pyramids.

First we start with a little philosophy.

"In the beginning God created the heavens and the earth...so God created man (this word means human unless the context specifically says otherwise. Only women get words devoted to only them.) **in His own image, in the image of God created He him; male and female created He them."** Genesis 1:27

"All things were made by Him and without Him was not anything made that was made." John 1:3

"God is love." John 4:8b

God made us and He loves us. He created this whole world for us to live in. He provided the perfect food to support us for all of eternity.

"And God said, Behold, I have given you every plant bearing seed, which is on the face of all the earth, and every tree, in the which is the fruit of a tree yielding seed. To you it shall be for meat (food). **And to every beast of the earth, and to every fowl of the**

air, and to every thing that creeps upon the earth, wherein there is life, I have given every green herb for meat (food)**: and it was so.**" Genesis 1:29

Everybody was originally a vegetarian, even the lions and vultures.

What happened? Adam and Eve disobeyed God. This brought death and disease into the world.

By the time of Noah, God told humans it was ok to eat meat. Many Creation scientists believe that some essential nutrient was leached from the soil during the flood and it is now only available through animal flesh. (Vitamin B_{12}?)

God commanded Israel to eat red meat once per year, minimum (Passover feast). I am not saying we should begin torching sheep again, but I have learned that there are often health reasons behind the commands that God gave His people, though the main reason for the commands were spiritual.

For example, Israel was to circumcise their baby boys (remove some of the skin from around the tip of the penis). Israel today still performs this ritual with nearly 100% of their sons while other western nations are moving away from doing this. Israel is the only modern western nation without a dramatic increase in cervical cancer. Could God have chosen this as the sign of membership in His nation to protect His daughters? Circumsition also drasticly reduces the rates of penial cancers, infections and unplesant oders.

God told Israel to wash after touching dead bodies. The doctors in the 1800's were "too advanced" to believe in such hocus-pocus. They would often perform an autopsy and then deliver a baby without even rinsing their hands. 50-80% of women who gave birth in a hospital died of post-birth infection. One doctor just rinsed his hands in plain water and cut his losses to less than 20%. Today, of course, they all scrub with disinfectant and now losses are less than 1%[11]. (Most women refused to go to the hospital to birth at this time. Homebirth with a midwife lost very few mothers or babies. This is still true today as you are already immune to the germs in your own home while you are not immune to the ones in a hospital where sick people go.)

There are more examples. The point is, I think God had a reason for choosing to command Israel to eat sheep at least once per year (instead of, say, carrots), and it may have been for their own health as well as for the spiritual significance of death being required to pay for our sin.

What is the first thing to do to be healthy? Well, we should think in the longest terms for health. You can't get longer than eternity. It is healthy to go to heaven. It is not healthy to go to hell. So how do you go to heaven? God's first command to Israel;

"Hear O Israel, the Lord your God is one God, (not 1,253 like the pagan nations believed... One. You only have to please One.) **And thou shalt love the Lord thy God with all thine heart, and with all thy soul, and with all thy might.** (With everything you've got. This leaves nothing for you to serve the un-satisfiable god

---

[11] America now loses 7 women per 100,000 live births. This is still much higher than, say Greece, who only loses 1 woman per 100,000 births, but birth is basicly safe in developed nations.

"Self" with. It is all God's and He is so much easier to please.)

And these words, which I command thee this day, shall be in thine heart; (If your heart is full of God's word, there is no room for fear, hatred, and worry) **and thou shalt teach them diligently unto thy children** (you don't really learn a thing to its full extent until you teach it to someone else, plus, this way your children are guaranteed to learn it) **and shalt talk of them when thou sittest in thine house, and when thou walkest by the way, and when thou liest down, and when thou risest up.** (Twenty-four hours a day. Well, ok, it doesn't say to teach them when you are asleep, but every waking minute. It isn't as easy to be a hypocrite with little eyes watching you all the time and listening to your every word)

And thou shalt bind them for a sign upon thine hand, and they shall be as frontlets between thine eyes. And thou shalt write them upon the posts of thy house, and on thy gates. (You will have them before your face at all times so you don't forget, and you must be literate to do this.)" Deuteronomy 6:4-9

Or as Jesus put it

"That whosoever believeth (an action verb) **in him should not perish, but have eternal life."** John 3:15

Giving your all to God is the healthiest thing you can do.

Studies have also shown that religious people have less depression and recover from serious illness faster and more completely. So belief in God is not only good for your eternal health, but for you right-now-health too.

Now for physical food.

Food can be divided into five categories;
- water,
- fruits and veggies,
- breads and grains,
- dairy, and
- meat.

Fruit and veggies are foods that come from the orchard and garden on our farm. This would include herbs, spices, maple trees, sugar cane and honey, because that is the best place for your beehives. We will put nuts and olives in this group for now. They are a little different nutritionally than most of what we call fruits and vegetables, but for ease of classifying we will lump them together. Also of course, apples, grapes, strawberries, carrots, tomatoes, spinach, pumpkin, etc. go here.

Grains and cereals come from the fields. This means wheat, corn, oats, rice, and oddly enough, potatoes (kind of "God's instant bread").

Meats come from the pasture. There are cows, pigs, sheep, deer (they jumped the fence to get the good pasture grass), chickens (special meat breeds. Not the egg layers), turkeys, ducks, and fish (in the pond). Meat is any food you have to take an animals life in order to eat.

Dairy comes from the barn. Cows and laying chickens aren't taken too far away from the barn because it would be too inconvenient to collect the product everyday. You do not kill an animal to eat dairy. A hen lays an egg everyday whether it has ever seen a rooster or not. It is just a natural part of her cycle. Eating an egg doesn't mean you kill a baby chick.

Your assignment, if you should choose to accept it, is to mentally put each food you eat this week into one of these classes.

Ingredients on labels are listed in the order of amount. On a cake's label, flour is the first ingredient so cake is a bread/grain product. (Second biggest ingredient is sugar, so you could call it a secondary fruit.) A candy bar usually has more sugar than anything else, so it is a fruit. Be careful, though. Manufacturers don't like to admit they put more sugar than anything else in their products. They will often use more than one kind of sugar in order to fool you. If you see a product with sugar, corn syrup, high fructose corn syrup, maltose, and fructose (in fact anything ending in -ose), you can be pretty sure there is more sugar than anything else in that product, even if none of those are the first ingredient.

For mixed foods, such as a burrito, you have to have more than one class. Let's see, a burrito would be bread because of the tortilla, meat because of the beef, dairy because of the cheese, and veggie/fruit because of the beans and salsa (tomatoes and peppers). Lasagna would be a bread/meat/cheese/fruit also. A hamburger is, well I guess it is the same if you have cheese on it. A tuna sandwich is a bread/meat. If you use mayo and pickles on it you can add dairy and fruit/veggie. Apple pie? Bread/fruit. You get the idea. This will help you to be aware of what you are actually eating. Bon 'appetite.

9. Nutrition Labels

What Does it all Mean?

The government mandates that all refined food products have a nutrition label. This is so you can make more informed choices.

Now the healthiest choices are foods that have no label at all (lettuce, apples, steak...). If we lived 200 years age, that is all that would be available to us (and the odds are very good we wouldn't have diabetes, heart disease, or cancer. Of course, we also wouldn't have Penicillin or indoor plumbing.) The truth is that we live in the 21st century and we do have to deal with processed food. So it is important that we learn to read labels so we can make wise choices.

The first thing the nutrition label shows you is how big a serving is. Be careful when comparing different brands of the same products. There is no standardization of what a serving is. I was comparing several foods the other day. One cereal listed a serving as one cup while the same cereal by a different manufacturer said a serving was ¾ of a cup. One brand of bread says a serving is one slice, while the next one on the shelf says it is two slices. One chocolate bar says a serving is 40 ounces, the next says it is 36, while the third says it's 12. Usually similar foods have the same serving size, but occasionally you need to do a little math (good thing all of our phones have calculators in them!)

The next thing listed is how many servings are in a container. Again, be careful. Some small cans of soup for example, have two servings (when everyone eats the whole thing in one sitting!).

The label then tells you how many calories in a serving, how many calories from fat, and what kinds of fat it has. Remember that mono-unsaturated is a GOOD fat (full of vitamins), poly-unsaturated is ok. Saturated fats from olive oil and butter are good, but all the trans-fats are very bad. Very few processed foods actually use olive oil or butter. They are too expensive.

The label then tells you how much cholesterol. This isn't really important as eating cholesterol isn't what makes your blood cholesterol rise. This info is there solely for PR purposes. Gummy bears and diet coke have no cholesterol, but that doesn't mean they are good for you.

Sodium is next. The RDA for sodium is 2400mg. This one adds up fast, but is really only a concern for those with sodium-sensitive high blood pressure.

Then we have total carbs followed by fiber and sugars. These "sugars" are not all cane sugar, but may mean some natural simple carbohydrates (though usually they mean added sugar). Fiber contains no calories itself, but is vitally important to your health.

Then we list protein.

Most labels list the percentage of RDA for several vitamins and minerals, but this isn't standardized so it may vary from label to label. The percentage is based on a diet of 2000 calories, so if you are an inactive woman[12], the nutrient would be a higher percentage of your diet

---

[12] It's not at all fair, but men naturally have a higher metabolism than women. Even if they are the same height, weight and activity level, the man will take more calories to just stay alive.An active woman needs 1800-2000calories a day. A man gets another 500-1000.

than listed. But if you are an active man it would be less than the percentage stated.

Below most nutrition labels is the ingredients list. The law demands that the ingredients are listed in order by weight present in the product.

So, in comparing two different products, the one with the lowest calories, sodium and fat but the highest protein and fiber is the better product.

What if two products are equal in most areas but, say, one is higher in protein and the other in fiber? Which one do you choose? It depends on what you are buying the product for. In my loaf bread I favor fiber since I don't rely on my bread to provide protein (bread is what I use to hold my protein so I can eat it neater). But in a snack bar, I favor the protein because the whole reason I use snack bars is for a quick protein fix. If you are having a problem with constipation, however, you may want to favor the higher fiber bars. This is an individual call.

RDA stands for "Recommended Dietary Allowance." This is the amount the government determined was necessary to prevent major deficiency disease but does not reflect the optimum amount for health. For example, the RDA for vitamin C is 60mg. This is what is necessary to prevent scurvy. However, researchers have discovered that those who take 500mg a day have far fewer colds and flues. The research is still ongoing to find the best levels for most nutrients.

10.   A Visit to the Orchard

Fruits, Nuts, and Sweets

"And God said, 'Let the earth bring forth grass, the herb yielding seed, and the fruit tree yielding fruit after his kind, whose seed is in itself, upon the earth:' and it was so." Genesis 1:11

Have you been putting all your food in one of the places on the farm? Good.

Let's start a more detailed tour in the orchard. While standing there, you are surrounded by trees of many different sizes, from the towering walnut and apple trees to the short, almost bushy plum and almond trees. Along the fence you see bushes and vines. Everything has fruits of many different colors; bright orange oranges; deep red apples, cherries and berries; purple plums and grapes; brownish-green nuts, and green apples, grapes and olives. Here is your first clue to eating healthy. All these good foods are VERY colorful. Cookies and chips are not (Yes, I know M&Ms and Skittles are colorful, too, but they don't count).

Those things we usually call fruit (berries, citrus, apples, grapes, etc.) are high in vitamin C, and most of the B's. If you don't get enough vitamin C you will get scurvy, a disease where your cells don't stick together so, if it is bad enough, you will bleed to death. Do your gums bleed? You may have a low level of scurvy beginning. Some believe lack of C can cause hardening of the arteries; Your arteries bleed because of a lack of C and grow stiff scar tissue.

Also, eating oranges has been shown to lower blood-pressure.

C has (finally) been proven to boost your immune system. It can help prevent colds and flues by making your natural army of sickness fighters stronger.

Most fresh fruits are high in fiber and water making it difficult to truly gorge yourself on them. They fill the tummy up quickly and the extra just "passes on through." More on fiber in a a later chapter.

Do you eat enough fruits? I don't, but I am working on it. Fresh is best. Straight from the tree or vine, but frozen, dried or canned in water are still good (frozen being best[13]). You should have at least three servings of fruit per day (more is better, and at least one should be citrus or berries for the vitamin C).

Oh goodness, here we go with the scales.

No. I want to make things easy. I'm too lazy to do otherwise. The amount you can comfortably hold in one hand is one serving. That would be one apple, one orange, half a cup or so of berries or grapes, or one cup of juice (though holding a cup of juice in your hand may be difficult unless you make sure you include the cup). Dried fruit gets half that amount for a serving because you took all the water out when you dried it. Smaller people (children) need fewer calories, but since they have smaller hands, their servings are automatically smaller.

---

[13] In fact, if your food is trucked in from long distances, frozen may be healthier than fresh. Frozen food is picked at the peek of ripeness and nutrient content and is immediately flash frozen, preserving almost all of its nutrients. "Fresh" fruit and veggies are picked before they are ripe and are often shipped long distances, ripening on the way (without roots to add nutrients from the ground though). They are often sprayed with wax to make them prettier. They may have been picked weeks before they reach your store, losing nutrients every minute of the way.

Trying to increase your fruit intake is not really hard. Have an orange with your breakfast. Add a handful of raisins or dried berries to your pancakes or fresh bread (just dump them in whether you use a mix or cook by scratch). Serve a can of fruit with supper, or keep the fruit bowl in the middle of the table for eveyone to munch on when the rest of the meal is done. Eat a sprig of grapes or a smoothie (3 cups of fruit, 1 cup of yogurt or juice, a dash of honey) for a snack.

Plan it in. Breakfast and supper aren't ready to eat until they have a fruit with them.

Don't change anything else for two weeks. Just add more fruit. Go slow, one fruit a day for a few days, then two per day for a few days and so on, so you don't shock your system.

How Sweet It Is

Sugars were in our orchard too. The bees need the trees to make honey, and this is where you would find the maple trees[14]. We will put the sugar cane and sugar beets here too.

"Pleasant words are as an honeycomb, sweet to the soul, and health to the bones." Proverbs 16:24

Honey

Honeybees go from flower to flower collecting the nectar which they process into honey in order to store it for later consumption[15]. A beekeeper gets the honey by blowing smoke into the hive, which puts the bees to sleep, and then scraping the honey out. He has to work

---

[14] Ok, not really. I would want mine in the pasture or front lawn because they are pretty, but that doesn't work with our health thing here.
[15] Sigh, Yes, Hubby, it's bee vomit.

fast so he can be done before the bees wake up. The honey is then run through a strainer and bottled. Most of the honey you buy in the store is pasteurized in order to kill any bacteria. Raw honey (UN-pasteurized) may contain trace amounts of some bacteria (so you don't EVER feed it to a child under one year of age) but it is actually very antiseptic. It is often used by herbalists to rub on a sore or injury to speed healing while preventing infection. It works because of the high sugar content, low pH and the presence of organic acids. Use it to treat cuts, scrapes and burns as well as to prevent scarring. Just rub a little honey on your wound. It will also cure a sore throat.

But of course that is not the point of this chapter. You want to know what kind of sweetener to put in your tea.

Raw honey contains:

B6	Calcium	Phosphorous
Thiamin	Copper	Potassium
Niacin	Iron	Sodium
Riboflavin	Magnesium	Zinc
Pantothenic Acid	Manganese	

It has natural antioxidants such as vitamin C. Using honey in your baked goods will keep them moist for a longer period of time than sugar. It is slightly acidic and, therefore, not conducive for bacterial growth.

Solomon said "Pleasant words are as an honeycomb, sweet to the soul, and health to the bones." He said 3000 years ago that pleasant words are as good for the bones as honey! The minerals contained in honey are the known bone builders of the world. I believe honey is the first choice, healthiest sweetener there is. It won't cause the blood glucose levels of many diabetics to rise like other sugars will. If at all possible use this in your cooking and teas.

Pasteurization destroys most of the nutrients in honey, but I still believe it is the healthiest.

Applesauce

Some people use applesauce in their cooking for a sweetener. Applesauce is made by peeling and coring apples; then cooking them down until they are a sauce. You could make your own. I intend to try someday.

When buying applesauce be sure to read the label. Many manufacturers add sugar. If you are looking for the healthiest sweetener, you do not want to use applesauce with sugar in it. The applesauce itself is high in fiber; as much as you will find in a slice of whole wheat bread or a serving of broccoli. A medium apple contains approximately 150 mg of potassium, almost 5% of your recommended daily value, and has just 70 calories and no sodium. This makes applesauce a great sweetener for baking.

Maple syrup

Real maple syrup is made by drilling a hole in the side of a maple tree and collecting the sap that runs out, then boiling the sap down until it is thick.

Maple syrup contains fewer calories and a higher concentration of a few minerals than honey, primarily manganese, and zinc.

Again, read the label when you go shopping. "Pancake syrup" is NOT the same thing as maple syrup. Pancake syrup is really corn syrup with "artificial maple flavorings" -what ever that is- added.

White grape juice

This sweetener is obtained by squeezing green grapes until you get all the juice out. I would assume what we buy in the store is pasteurized (heated at a high temperature until all the bacteria is killed). It may be easier for babies to digest than other juices since it has a simpler sugar structure. Red grape juice has all the same benefits as wine without any of the bad effects of alcohol. It contains the same powerful disease-fighting antioxidants, called flavonoids that are believed to give wine many of its heart-friendly benefits. Good stuff.

All the above sweeteners can be grown and processed on a small farm.

Agave Nectar

Agave is the plant Tequila is made from. However, the unfermented juice is 1.5 times sweeter than sugar, milder flavored than honey (with the darker varieties resembling maple syrup), and slower to digest. Many diabetics can use it when they can't use sugar or honey. It is, however, a processed food. You can't make it on your farm.

Concentrated fruit juice

I have heard of people using frozen orange or apple juice to replace all or part of the sweet in a recipe. This would give all the same benefits as the fresh juices as long as it doesn't contain sugar.

Sugar (cane or beet sugar)

Sugar is made by harvesting sugar canes or sugar beets, squeezing the juice out, dehydrating the juice, then bleaching what is left until it is pure white. Though you could grow the sugar cane and sugar beets on your farm, you can't make white sugar at home, especially from the beets which take more processing than the canes.

I think table-sugar is one of the greatest health evils of all time. Not too long ago doctors actually recommended people eat table-sugar. They don't do that anymore. Want to know why? There are actually more studies linking table-sugar to heart disease and cancer than there are linking fat to either (there just is no "fat" public relations firm, while the sugar PR group is very powerful).

America's consumption of table sugar has increased by 500% in the last twenty years while their consumption of fats has gone down. Yet heart disease continues to rise.

Table-Sugar raises the insulin level of the blood. The body uses insulin to keep blood-sugar at a constant and safe level. Insulin also promotes the storage of fat, so that when you eat sweets high in table-sugar, you're making it easier to gain weight, as well as risking a dibetic reaction. Complex carbohydrates (breads, fruit, and veggies) tend to be absorbed more slowly, lessening the impact on blood-sugar levels.

Table-sugar inhibits the release of growth hormones, which in turn depresses the immune system. This is not something you want to take place if you want to avoid disease of any kind.

Our disease fighting white-blood cells also need vitamin C to kill bacteria and viruses. Table-sugar changes into glucose in the digestive tract. Glucose is very similar to vitamin C in structure but not at all similar in action. So when our white blood cells go to absorb vitamin C, they will take in glucose leaving no room for sufficient amounts of C.

It only takes a blood sugar value of 120 to reduce the virus-killing power of our cells by 75%. So when you eat table sugar, think of your immune system slowing down to a crawl.

The cause of all disease is at the cellular level. Feed and care for the cells correctly and you will prevent disease, from the common cold to cancer. Table-sugar harms the cells at the most basic levels.

Table-sugar has been observed to worsen asthma, mood swings, personality changes, mental illness, nervous disorders, Diabetes, heart disease, gallstones, arthritis, and a whole lot more.

It takes enzymes, vitamins and minerals to digest sugar. Unprocessed sugars, such as fruit, come with the things necessary for that digestion. Table-sugar has had them processed out; so it steals nutrients from the body in order to digest it. When these vitamin stores are too low our bodies can't use cholesterol and fatty acids correctly. This makes the blood levels of cholesterols and triglycerides too high because our bodies can't take them out of the blood to use them. This raises your risk of disease from these chemicals being in the wrong places, (because your body doesn't have what it needs to clean them out properly). The American Dietetic Association and American Diabetic Association agree that sugar consumption in America is one of the 3 major causes of degenerative disease.

Cancer's preferred food has been shown in laboratories to be glucose (That is what they feed cancer in the Petri dish to keep it alive so they can find a cure for it. Hmmmm). When you eat table sugar your body turns it into glucose thus providing more food for any cancer cells in your body.

So, table sugars work like a secondary poison in your body. They rob you of the vitamins you already have in your system, prevent the absorption of any you might be eating, gum up the digestive process to prevent your body from kicking bad stuff out and then feed the very cancers that will kill you.

Oh, and they will rot your teeth. My sister-in-law, who is a dentist, says one of her teachers would not allow his children to brush their teeth or eat sugar. He showed the class x-rays of his grown children's mouths. Not a single cavity! She watched a video of an x-ray of a gorilla eating. As long as he ate natural food you could see the normal juices flowing down around and out of his teeth. When he was fed table sugar, the fluids began flowing the other way, pulling bacteria up into his teeth.

Avoid sugar, corn syrup, high fructose corn syrup, glucose, and sucrose (all names for refined sugar) as much as you possibly can. In fact, any ingredient that ends in –ose is some sort of sugar.

The only good thing I can say about table-sugar is that because nothing but cancer can grow in it, if you cut yourself you can coat the wound in sugar and it will kill the bacteria just like honey will. Just don't eat it.

Table sugar does have the advantage that it is the cheapest of all home sweeteners, as well as much easier to clean up if it spills than, say, honey. Those factors do need to be weighed in when making your choices.

Table-sugar is an addictive substance. You will probably have withdrawal symptoms if you go off of it cold turkey; headaches, mood swings, fatigue, etc. They should last about two weeks. Than you should feel better than ever.

Corn syrup (Caro syrup)

Same as above except made from corn and not as dehydrated. This is classified as a white sugar, except it is now suspected that it messes up our hormones responsible for weight regulation and immune system functions worse than table sugar.

Dextrose

Known as glucose or corn sugar. It is made from cornstarch. See above.

Confectioner's sugar (powdered sugar)

Table sugar mixed with cornstarch and pounded to a powder.

Raw sugar or Turbinado

Unbleached, refined sugar. Better than table sugar, but not by much.

Sugar alcohols

Metabolized more slowly than sugar (though with only three calories per gram insead of four) or just passed on through undigested: sorbitol, mannitol, xylitol and some others that are less common. They are derived from fruit.

These are used in chewing gum and toothpaste because they are not converted into sugar in the mouth though they taste sweet. Xylitol has even been shown to figh tooth decay and help remineralize the teeth. On going research is suggesting they don't affect blood sugar but do cause tummy problems (gas, bloating, someimes diarreha) in some people, especially when you eat too much of them.

Molasses

Ever wonder where all the vitamins God put in the sugar cane go to after man is through making sugar? That is what we call molasses. Molasses is separated from raw sugar during processing. Darker molasses and blackstrap molasses are superior in providing small amounts of some vitamins and minerals. This byproduct is high in:

Iron	Copper,	Potassium
Calcium	Manganese	Magnesium

Use it in your baking for a very distinct yet healthy flavor. Generally in America though, it is fed to cattle instead of people.

Brown sugar

Sugar crystals colored with molasses syrup. It has a few more minerals from the molasses than the white stuff, but not enough to call it "healthy."

Rapadura

Dehydrated Cane Sugar Juice. It is relatively unprocessed yet tastes a lot like sugar. You can easily over do it like sugar though.

Fructose or laevulose

Used as a table-sugar substitute. Fructose does not require insulin to get into the liver and body cells. It is processed from fruit juice. It does not have as many bad effects as sugar but is still missing the life-giving vitamins, minerals, and fiber of the fruit itself or natural sweeteners. You can't make it on your farm.

Saccharine (Sweet 'N Low)

OK I am going to admit something here; I have a very strong distrust of man-made foods. All artificial sweeteners are man made in the laboratory. I just don't think we can create things like food without messing it up somehow. If "tar parts" were good for us and God loves His children then why didn't He make them available before the late 1800's? Why did He deny all those people before that time, the pleasure of this sweet? This belief taints anything I say about artificial any-things.

I am finding conflicting reports on saccharine. First of all, a man accidentally invented it after running experiments on tar and not washing his hands enough before eating. Doesn't that sound appetizing?

I can't find information that explains in English (instead of scientist-eze) what exactly saccharine is. The little pink packet of stuff is a mix of dextrose (corn sugar), cream of tartar (grape extract), silicate (major component of sand), and saccharine. But no one seems to want to really explain what that last thing is besides "sweet."

The famous study that showed saccharine to cause cancer in rats was flawed. They fed those rats what would be the equivalent of sixty pounds per day to a human. I think if you ate sixty pounds of ANYTHING everyday it might cause cancer (if you didn't explode first!)

However, there are some hints here and there that those that drink as many as two saccharin sodas a day do have a slightly higher risk of bladder cancer. There is no hard evidence, though. If you are diabetic or Hypoglycemic and can not tolerate honey (some diabetics and hypoglycemic can and some can't) then you could use small amounts of Sweet N Low.

Aspartame (Equal, NutraSweet)

"A nonessential amino acid, C4H7NO4, found especially in young sugar cane and sugar-beet molasses."

Ok, so Equal comes originally from plants, but then it is totally changed on a molecular level in the laboratory to make it indigestible (thus it adds no calories).

"Some of the scientists and others working with the chemicals in the factory when Equal first came on the market contracted brain cancer, others simply disappeared when they began 'getting sick' – this was relayed to me by a former employee whose name I can no longer remember" Quote from an anti-aspartame website.

I found many studies saying aspartame is very, very, bad. The few that say otherwise can easily be discredited since the scientists that gave the good reports went to work for the NutraSweet Corporation shortly after the publication of their supportive reports.

Some of the symptoms of aspartame poisoning include: Headaches/Migraines, (I get these when I drink too many diet sodas), Weight gain(! Isn't that what we are trying to prevent by drinking the stuff in the first place?) plus

Dizziness	Irritability	Anxiety attacks
Seizures	Tachycardia	Slurred Speech
Nausea	Insomnia	Loss of taste
Numbness	Vision Problems	Tinnitus
Muscle spasms	Hearing Loss	Vertigo
Rashes	Heart palpitations	Memory loss
Depression	Breathing difficulties	Joint Pain
Fatigue		

I have found this list in many places (though each author words it slightly differently of course) over the course of many years.

Aspartame metabolizes into a poison, (Formaldehyde!), and other dangerous chemicals (despite the claims of the manufacturers to the contrary). It is believed that it can trigger or worsen the following conditions:

Brain tumors	Parkinson's	Fibromyalgia
Arthritis	Disease	Diabetes
Multiple	Alzheimer's	Thyroid
sclerosis	Mental	Disorders
Epilepsy	retardation	
Chronic fatigue	Lymphoma	
syndrome	Birth defects	

Aspartame is not sweet in itself. Equal Company puts Dextrose (sugar) and maltodextrin into it so that it tastes sweet. NutraSweet is a brain drug that stimulates your brain so you think that the food you're eating tastes sweet. If you pay attention you'll notice that when using NutraSweet, everything you eat at the same time also tastes sweet! (Try this experiment: take a bite of hamburger, chewing slowly paying attention to how sweet it tastes. Then take a big drink of diet soda. Wait a few minutes to give it a chance to get to your brain. Take another bite of hamburger and see if it tastes sweeter than the first bite.) This brain-stimulating causes you to crave even more carbohydrates, especially sweet things. So you won't lose weight using aspartame.

Oh, and the chemical it turns into, Formaldehyde, is thought to cause cancer. Do I need to say more?

Splenda/Sucrolose

Splenda is made by fusing two molecules of sucrose (table sugar) and three molecules of chlorine (a poison used to kill bacteria). Some scientists say Splenda has more in common with DDT (bug poison) than with food on a molecular level. The manufacture's own short-term studies showed that sucralose, (the chemical name for Splenda), caused shrunken thymus glands and enlarged livers and kidneys in rodents. Observational evidence shows that there are side effects of Splenda, including:

Skin Rashes/Flushing
Panic-Like Agitation
Dizziness
Numbness
Muscle Aches
Headaches
Intestinal Cramping
Bladder Issues

Reduced Growth Rate
Decreased Red Blood
Cell Count
Extension of Pregnancy
Miscarriage
Decreased Birth And
Placental Weights
Diarrhea

No one can say to what degree Splenda is affecting us. This chemical is still too new to know for sure. Many believe it to be the healthiest of the artificial sweeteners (earning an endorsement from the Center for Science in the Public Interest), but that isn't really saying much.

Stevia/Rabina

A sweet powder (rabina) made from a South American herb (stevia), or a liquid tincture made from the raw herb. Gram for gram, it is 30-300 times sweeter than sugar (depending on who you ask) with few or no calories. I have some of the dehydrated plant and it is very sweet to eat straight (with a slight grassy after taste) and I have a friend who is going to try to grow some in her vegetable garden. Over all, the least processed of the "artificial" sweeteners, though I'm not sure it shouldn't be classified as a natural sweetener instead.

Stevia has been used by natives of Paraguay for at least 400 years and in Japan for 30-40 (where it makes up 40% of all sweeteners used).

Stevia has:

- Possible positive effect on triglycerides, cholesterol and obesity
- anti-inflammatory effect
- may help diarrhea
- negligible effect on blood glucose (i.e. safe for diabetics)
- used in South America to actually treat diabetes, but few studies to support this claim
- may lower blood pressure
- may treat heartburn
- may improve skin rashes like eczema and eliminate dandruff [16]

Some European studies have shown an affect on the male reproductive system from use of this product. When male rats were fed **high doses** (up to 1000 times/pound of body weight than what any human would eat) of stevioside for 22 months, sperm production was reduced and when female hamsters were fed **large** amounts of a derivative of stevioside called steviol, they had fewer and smaller offspring. These studies are old, though, and many consider them poorly done.

"In the laboratory, steviol can be converted into a compound, which may promote cancer by causing mutations in the cells' genetic material."

---

[16] http://www.kitchenstewardship.com/2011/09/22/a-sweet-sweet-summer-what-are-the-facts-on-stevia/#tPb65EXBKDLkQpFw.99

"Very large amounts of stevioside can interfere with the absorption of carbohydrates in animals and disrupt the conversion of food into energy within cells."

On the other hand, in another study *"The rats who received the stevioside weighed less than those in the control group. Considering stevioside has no calories, this makes sense. When the organs and tissues of the rats were examined under a microscope, there was almost no difference between those who were given stevia and those who were not. One interesting difference, however, was that the females who took stevioside had a decreased incidence of* **breast tumors**, *while the males displayed a lesser incidence of* **kidney damage**. *The researchers state, 'It is concluded that stevioside is not carcinogenic in rats under the experimental conditions described.'* "[17]

And

"Acute toxicity was not demonstrated when separate 2 g/kg doses were administered to mice by oral intubation, indicating that a concentrated extract of stevia is less than 1/10 as toxic (acute) as caffeine."[18] (They found absolutely no traces of cancer or any other problems.)

Some claim those in Paraguay use Stevia as a contraceptive. If this is true, it isn't a very good one since they have double-digit birth rates (10 or more babies per woman where in America and Europe birthrates are, for example, 1.9-1.2 babies per woman.)

---

[17] Excerpted from: "The Stevia Cookbook," copyright 1999 by Ray Sahelian, MD and Donna Gates
[18] Gras Affirmation Petition, Stevia leaves, presented on behalf of the American Herbal Products Association, April 23, 1992

That is a lot of "can" and "may." We just don't know yet.

I do know that Stevia is perfetly natural in its unprocessed state, but then so is poison Hemlock (one of the most poisoness plants in the world). What is available in the stores is mildly processed.

I am cautious but hopeful about Stevia since it is a direct creation of God and not a bunch of chemicals from a laboratory. It is logical to me that it could actually be good for you. I hope we will know soon.

The bottom line: If you use Stevia sparingly, it probably isn't a great threat to you; might even be good for you. But if Stevia were processed and marketed widely and used in diet sodas (which Americans drink by the gallon), it probably would loose all it's good features, though it might still be better than any of the other white powders. We simply don't know enough yet. That's why there needs to be more testing.

<u>Acesulfame Potassium/ Ace-K</u>

200 times sweeter than sugar, this is the sweetener in Coke Zero. It is too new to know its affects yet, but pelimanary studies say it may cause breast and lung tumors and may cause thyroid problems, but all we have so far are animal studies. We don't know the long term affect of it on humans.

<u>Neotame</u>

Manufactured by the same people that give us Aspartame, this sweetener is chemically very similar. Neotame, however, can tolerate high temperatures without the chemical dangers of Aspartame. It is 8,000 times sweeter than sugar, meaning you need very, very little. This has also been approved by the Center for

Science in the Public Interest . Since it has only been approved since 2002 we don't really know its long term affect either.

You know, I think Americans just eat too many sweet things. It seems that we have grown to think everything has to be sweet (and sugar cravings are a symptom of diabetes). Did you know that some manufacturers even put sugar in their sweet corn? Maybe we should just look for ways to wake up our other taste buds; ways to enjoy other flavors such as salt, good-bitters, and sours and less sweet.

Conclusion- Use those sweets that God made if at all possible. The more man messes in things the more he messes them up.

"There is a way which seemeth right unto a man, but the end thereof are the ways of death." Proverbs 14:12, Proverbs 16:25

Just like in your life. If you try to make all our decisions based on your knowledge or what human experts say, you will mess up your whole life. If you base your decisions on what God says, everything will work out fine.

"And we know that all things work together for good to those who love God, to those who are the called according to His purpose." Romans 8:28

So, when choosing something sweet to eat, pick a fresh, whole fruit. Frozen is a close second choice (and in some cases, beats out fresh). Dried or canned are your third choices. Try using pure frozen fruit juice or apple sauce to sweeten your baking.

After that, raw honey is the most natural sweetener (you can and do eat it straight from the hive).

After honey would come maple syrup, molasses (what is leftover from processing sugar), or probably raw Stevia.

Then brown sugar.

Raw sugar is better than white, and I really believe white is better than the chemicals.

The exception to all this is those with sensitivities to real sugars, such as diabetics and hypoglycemics. They may not be able to tolerate any real sugars of any kind. For these people, I am glad we have the artificial sugars for very occasional treats. Pick Splenda, or Sweet N Low over NutraSweet. I (pre-diabetic) actually rotate which artificial sweeteners I use to reduce the risk of any of them.

At home I use honey, maple syrup, raw sugar and stevia. In restaurants I use the pink stuff in my tea. This should greatly reduce the risk of any adverse effects of any of them.

Favor the fruit if you can though because they are much healthier. God gave us these wonderful, ready-made desserts for our own enjoyment. He just added enough nutrients to make them healthy too.

<u>The Rest of the Orchard</u>

"And I have given you a land for which you did no work for, and cities which you didn't build, and you live in them. You eat from vineyards and olive yards which you didn't plant." Joshua 24:13

There are some trees in our orchard that are not in the same category as other fruits nutritionally. Avocados, coconuts, nuts and olives are high fat foods, though they are the fruit of the tree (cucumbers are the fruit of the vine, for comparison. "Fruit" is the seed bearing organ.) They are not in the same class as the other fruits (they don't have as much natural sugar), but are good treats. They are high in fat, but it is good fat.

Yes, there is such a thing as good fat. These fats have fat soluble vitamins (such as E) and are easily digested by the body. They help your hair, skin, and nails to be shinny and strong – prettier. They have not been linked to heart disease like some fats have.

Nuts, and to a lesser degree olives, are also high in protein, so when you eat them only some of the calories come from the expensive fat type of calories. Aim for adding one handful a day to your diet. You can eat them straight or throw them into your cooking, (stir fry, baked goods, some meat dishes and put them on salads instead of croutons).

Check the label on any prepared coconut you eat, though. Many manufacturers add sugar.

Olives are a special fruit. They are very high in fat and many scientists originally thought they were very bad for you because they look like the bad fats on a molecular level (saturated). But people in the Mediterranean region eat large amounts of olive products and almost never have heart disease. What gives? Turns out the human body thinks olives are carbohydrates! So you use them like a fat, but digest them like a carb. Olive oil is one of the best fats around. As much as you can, use olive oil or butter (more on that later). Extra virgin olive oil is simply the oil that is squeezed out of the olive (the same as orange juice is what comes out of an orange when you squeeze it). No processing. (Watch out for "extra light olive oil." It doesn't have as strong of a flavor, but it has been processed and lost the benefits of the extra virgin stuff).

Nut oils are your second best fats to add to your cooking because they are processed the same way as olive oil.

Same for canola oil.

Veggie oil, soy bean oil and corn oil are cooked and bleached. Their molecular structure is actually changed (hydrogenated – pumped full of hydrogen gas) so they will not spoil as fast. These are the ones that clog your arteries.

Avoid them.

Read labels.

Once again, eat the foods as close to how God made them as possible when you have a choice; olive oil instead of Crisco oil, fresh nuts instead of chocolate coated nuts, fruit off the tree instead of fruit pie, a spoon of honey instead of a Twinkie. God knew what He was doing when He made this world and provided these foods for us.

11.   The Garden

Vegetables and Herbs

"And God said, Behold, I have given you every plant bearing seed, which is upon the face of all the earth, and every tree that has seed bearing fruit. To you it shall be for food."

Genesis 1:29

In our garden we find the veggies and herbs. I like to picture my garden as a series of raised beds. Just a personal thing. I think that looks prettier than traditional rows.

Here we find lettuce, greens, tomatoes, cucumbers, squash, broccoli, celery, eggplant, oh, I could go on and on. Let's talk about categories.

The "Green leafies" such as Romaine lettuce, and spinach, are high in vitamin A. (I don't like my greens cooked at all. I prefer them in a salad. However, many like them lightly sautéed in just a touch of butter). This vitamin is good for your eyes, skin, and blood clotting ability. They are also high in calcium (two cups of raw spinach has the same calcium as a cup of milk).

The darker the green the more vitamins and minerals. Iceberg ("normal" lettuce) doesn't have very much more than water and fiber and not much of those, so choose the loose leaf, dark green lettuce when you can.

Did you know that Dandelion greens (the leaf, not the stem) are in the same class? Dandelions:

Support Digestion   Reduce Swelling And
                                     Inflammation

Treat Viruses	Gout
Jaundice	Eczema
Edema	Acne

and are very high in calcium. This common "weed" is often used as a medicinal herb and is incredibly high in vitamins (often higher than spinach). Yes, instead of poisoning the weeds in your front lawn, you should go eat them!

Umm, you may want to pick them and take them inside. The neighbors might think you have flipped if you go grazing.[19]

You should have at least two servings of greens per day. A serving of veggies is the same size as a serving of fruit (one hand full), so a big salad has two or more servings of greens. Have you ever tried fresh spinach greens on your hamburger instead of iceberg lettuce? Tastes a lot like lettuce but with WAY more vitamins. Do a little research and experiment!

Reds: Tomatoes are relatively high in vitamin C and can count as part of a citrus serving. And when they are cooked, they actually increases their cancer and heart-disease fighting chemicals. So enjoy plenty of spaghetti sauce, pizza sauce, ketchup, salsa and any other tomato based products you want.

Red peppers are higher in vitamin C than green. In fact, take any color over green if you can afford it because of higher vitamins, though the green bell peppers are packed, too.

---

[19] I am only hitting the high spots on vitamins and minerals. These foods have many, many more nutrients that I am not discussing.

Other peppers are high in vitamin C and the "hot" increases your metabolism and supreses your appetite (for several hours afterward!)

Orange veggies, such as carrots and pumpkins, contain Beta Carotene, which the body converts into vitamin A. Beta Carotene is also used for many cellular functions. In fact, all the things we think about when we think of veggies (except corn, peas, and potatoes. They are in the bread and grain class nutritionally) are very high in A and B vitamins, calcium and other minerals, and fiber. You should have at least three servings per day total, and as with the fruit, more is better. Frozen may actually be better than fresh since frozen veggies are picked at the peak of ripeness and flash frozen, preserving all the nutrients. Fresh produce is often picked before it is ripe and shipped to the stores. That squash you are looking at may have been off the vine as long as two weeks, losing nutrients every hour since it was picked.

Let's see, a big green salad with tomato, red sweet pepper slices, cucumber, carrot slices, celery chunks, drizzled with olive oil and lemon juice or topped with salsa, and with chopped nuts and raisins. Sounds good! Hmmm, maybe I had better go eat some lunch.

Herbs are used for four main purposes: food, medicines, flavorings, and decorations (for the eyes and the nose.)

Many things we call herbs (Alfalfa, Dandelion, Raspberry leaf, etc.) are actually foods equal, or superior, to the more common veggies on our dinner tables such as iceberg lettuce, broccoli, green beans, etc. They can be eaten freely without worry.

As far as **medicines** go, I believe that God didn't leave humanity with no relief for common ailments for thousands of years. He has provided help in the form of garlic to boost the immune system, Aloe Vera and Plantain to sooth cuts, burns and skin abrasions, Feverfew to reduce fever and calm headaches, Dandelion roots to help blood sugar issues, Peppermint for stomach upset, Chamomile to sooth the nerves, and on and on. I have only begun to study this area, but am amazed at the things our God has provided to all of humanity throughout the ages. Gee, you would think He cared about us or something.[20]

Now I am not saying we shouldn't ever use modern medicines. They have their place (such as when my daughter broke her arm) and I am thankful for them. But many times we are too quick to look to human doctors as if they were divine.

"I have purple spots on my hair, so I will see a doctor. He says I should take medicine X three times a day, so that must be what I need"

"Gee Doc, why does my arm twitch now that I am taking medicine X?"

"Oh you need medicine Y to counteract that."

"Medicine Y gave me hives on the bottom of my feet."

"Then you need medicine Z, too" and on it goes until we are all a walking Pharmacy.

The truth is, doctors are not required to take nutrition in college. They are required to take

---

[20] See "The ABC Herbal," "The How To Herb Book," anything by Shonda Parker, and many other good herb books out there. The Easlings at http://thebulkherbstore.com have a wide selection of herbs for sale and a great deal of information available for free on their website.

Pharmaceuticals (pill classes- most medical schools are supported in large part by donations from Pharmaceutical companies.). Doctors are human, make mistakes, and are limited in knowledge. When they hear a complaint they immediately think of what they have heard to solve it. But all pharmaceuticals have side effects. Just some more than others.

Here is the wise way to deal with medicines; If you have an ailment, try changing your lifestyle first to take care of it (eat more fruits and veggies, exercise more, reduce your stress, etc. No negative side effects whether it works or not.)

If that doesn't work, check out the most natural treatments (herbs) you can find (few side effects if taken in recommended doses. More is not always better in herbs anymore than it is in pharmaceuticals. More than the recommended dose of Aspirin will harm your body in stead of help it. Same for Feverfew and other medicinal herbs).

If they don't work, try over the counter medications (some side effects).

And if that fails see your doctor for a prescription (more side affects).

Only if that doesn't work consider surgery (potentially fatal).

This of course doesn't apply to emergencies such as breaking your leg or having a heart attack (no amount of Dandelion Salad will fix a broken arm). America has the best emergency care on the planet and you don't want to be anywhere else if you need immediate attention than in one of our doctor's offices. But for lesser complaints, it only makes sense to use that cure that will provide relief with the least amount of harmful side effects.

Many of the herbs used can and are used for **flavorings in cooking**. All cooking herbs (Garlic, Onions, Peppers, Rosemary, Thyme, Sage, ginger, etc.) provide at least some vitamins, so use them freely. Generally, the fresher the better. The mojority of them are very anti-microbial and will help infections and most ailments.

The **decorative herbs** are good for the soul. God made us to enjoy being surrounded by beauty. We need that in our heart, so pretty flowers, interesting grasses and all the sweet smelling things in the world are good for you even if you only put them on your table instead of in your food. Edith Schaeffer in *The Hidden Art of Homemaking* says "If you can only afford two loaves of bread or a loaf of bread and a bouquet of flowers, buy the flowers." I agree. Don't starve your soul for those things God has made for our pleasure.

Did you know some flowers are edible? Roses, Violets, Dandelions (the flower, not the stem. The stem is poisonous), Imagine what a pretty salad that would make? Or a stir fry with flowers, broccoli, cauliflower, fresh green beans, bell peppers, maybe a few potatoes or yams, some nuts, and water with a dash of olive oil. Yummm. These are all very high in vitamins. Just make sure they were not grown with any pesticides or herbicides. You don't want to poison yourself.

One major benefit of a high plant diet is that veggies and fruit are higher in fiber. The shear bulk of these foods physically fill up your stomach without providing more calories. You eat more veggies; you feel fuller but are taking in fewer calories. They are harder to eat (you have to actually chew them) so your meals last longer and are more emotionally satisfying (besides chomping uses more calories than gulping). You could even munch on them between meals without jeopardizing your diet. You feel like you are cheating but you aren't.

God wants what is best for us. That is why He has made the rules He has made. He knows what is best far better than we do. He provided a variety of foods in a variety of colors and textures for Adam and Eve to eat. I am not saying we should all quit eating meat. In fact, for reasons I will go into later, I believe we need meat. But most Americans need to eat way more fruits and veggies than we do.

12. Field Crops

Breads, Grains, and Potatoes

"And God said, Behold, I have given you every plant bearing seed, which is upon the face of all the earth, and every tree which has fruit with a seed. To you it shall be for food." Genesis 1:29

Fields are for crops which need to be grown in large amounts and must be replanted every year. We will grow wheat, oats, corn, rice, and potatoes. You could put peas and beans here as well as in the vegetable garden.

The wheat kernel, though small, is one of the biggest sources of nutrients in the world. It has carbs and protein, fiber, minerals and vitamins. Straight from the plant, the wheat kernel is sort of like "God's vitamin pack." Too bad humans can't leave it alone.

The first thing we do to the wheat kernel is to remove the outer coating called the bran (the equivalent of the shell on an egg, the skin of an apple or the brown part of an almond). This is the entire amount of fiber in wheat.

Gone.

Now the resulting bread is nice and white and fluffy. Until that is, it arrives in your colon. Then it is like paste. The bran is what keeps it "going on through" like it is supposed to. Fiber also dissolves into your blood stream and scrapes your arteries clean, just like a broom on your kitchen floor. It is necessary for health. One doctor has stated that more than half of America's common ailments could be cured if people would just eat more fiber.

How do you tell if you have enough fiber? Well...(I know this is gross) Fiber floats. Your bowel movements will float. You should also have at least one bowel movement per day (many believe you should have one for each meal you eat.) This is the sign that every thing is going through as it should be. The constipation medications you buy in the store are mostly made up of the bran the manufacturers removed from your bread as well as certain herbs that are high in fiber. As I have been saying, fiber is available in fruit, veggies, legumes and whole grain bread products.

Next, we remove the germ. This is the part of the kernel that the baby plant would grow from (the equivalent of the yolk of an egg or the core of the apple). It is where more than twenty-four known nutrients are stored. When we cut that part off; "bye-bye vitamins."

Why would manufacturers do this? Simple. Bread with no nutrients can not support life so the bread will not be invaded by the bacteria that would cause it to spoil and mold. Less spoilage equals greater profits.

Besides, most people think it tastes better. Of course the problem that comes up is that it can't support human life either. The solution? Add seven vitamins into the flour and call it enriched. This "enriched" flour is listed on labels as flour, white flour, wheat flour, and enriched flour. It doesn't really matter what it is called. It is the nutritional equivalent of eating just the white part of an egg. White flour is little more than sugar, nutritionally.

Then, in most cases, the flour is bleached; chemically treated to make it snow white instead of its natural creamy white. Honestly, if you saw unbleached flour by itself you would probably think it was pure white, it is so light. It isn't until you get it next to bleached flour that you can tell the unbleached is creamy colored.

There are two different chemicals used to bleach flour (both used at the same time). My main objection is that one of these chemicals is the same one used to give laboratory rats Diabetes in order to find a cure for the disease. Hmmm.

An island in the pacific was discovered to have a large amount of a valuable metal. Before the discovery, the people grew all their own food and ate nothing refined. Missionaries and doctors who went there to evaluate their health reported the people as being very healthy. No signs of diseases. After the discovery, they began importing their food and living a life of leisure (sale of the metal made them all rich). Today they have a nearly 100% Diabetes rate.

On the Mexican/ American border, there is a tribe of Indians. Half the tribe lives in Mexico and half in America. Both live in the same region and come from the same genetic stock. The Mexican half of the tribe still eats the way their ancestors did; they grow their food themselves. They have little illness, no obesity, and no Diabetes. The American branch lives a modern American lifestyle eating all refined foods. They all have Diabetes.

You will find this repeated over and over again all over the world; Natural unrefined diet (plus the exercise that comes from growing your own food) equals little disease. Add refined food (and I am sure the great couch-potato-maker known as TV) and suddenly you have high rates of disease, especially Diabetes.

It happens every time.

I really think this chemical used to bleach the flour is a major factor in this phenomenon, though probably not the only one (the mumps vaccine is known to increase the rate of diabetes).

The only way to make sure you don't get any of this depleted flour is to only eat what you make yourself or only buy products labeled 100% whole grain or 100% whole wheat. I realize this is nearly impossible in this society, but most of us could eat more whole grains than we do. And manufacturers are beginning to realize that some will buy more from them if they use the whole grain. (There is a new breed of wheat out there that is very light in color and flavor while still being the complete, whole grain. Inside of cereal, it is almost indistinguishable from white flour. Many cereal manufacturers are now using this wheat so they can make moms happy.)

Whenever you have a choice, pick whole wheat or whole grain breads, crackers, pasta, breading and cereal. Compare the labels though. Some manufacturers add so much sugar to their bread to try to get your business that they destroy all the benefits of having the whole grain.

Wheat is best eaten after having certain enzymes in it neutralized. However, God, in His wisdom, made the best way to neutralize those enzymes. You see, in order to make wheat soft enough and full enough of yeast to rise, you must soak it for several hours in water and an acid base (at least you did until the invention of modern dry yeast). This soaking happens to also be the way to neutralize the bad enzymes making the vitamins more available and the flour more digestible.

All that I have said could be applied to rice also. Most of the rice we eat is "polished" so that it is nice and bright white. Rice with its bran still on is tan colored and a little chewier than white rice. Takes a little longer to cook, also. Many Asians suffered a great deal from Thiamin deficiency when this polishing technology was invented. Their governments now dust white rice with Thiamin powder to alleviate this. This doesn't make up for the missing bran, though.

Eating a variety of grains is a good way to get a multitude of different vitamins. Each kind of grain has a different balance. Corn is actually a grain, not a veggie as most of us use it. It has lots of complex carbs (slow-to-digest bread sugars) and some amino acids that are low in other grains.

If you eat a legume (beans, peas, or peanuts) with your grain product you are getting a complete protein (read the label on your peanut butter though. Most brands have had the good peanut fat removed and bad hydrogenated fat put in; then they douse it in sugar). You see, your body needs certain amino acids in order to function right.

Any animal protein has all of them. Grains only have some and legumes only have some. But legumes are short where grains tend to be high and grains are short where legumes are high. If you eat the two together, you have the same amino acids you have in a steak or a cup of milk. I have experimented with adding bean flour to my whole grain breads. This makes a slice of bread even richer in nutrients. Sometime read Ezekiel 4:9. God gives him a recipe (unfortunately without the amounts) for bread that Ezekiel was to live on for more than a year. It included grains and legumes. It would have had everything his body needed for the very inactive time he had ahead of him.

Nuts, though raised as a fruit, are a legume nutritionally. They are high in protein and "good" fats.

Studies have shown that people who eat lots of nuts have greater success maintaining weight and avoiding heart disease.

Potatoes are kind of like God's quick bread. Nutritionally they are high in vitamin C, potassium and carbohydrates. They are better for you than white bread, though there are more vitamin-rich breads you could be eating. I really think though, (unless you have a sensitivity) the biggest damage is the extra things most people do to their potatoes. Fast food restaurants deep fry them in fat; Hydrogenated veggie fat at that. All the vitamins are cooked out and just about all that is left is the veggie fat (which is the type of fat linked to heart disease.) Now, the same potato cooked in butter or beef fat is a whole different story!

Extra sour cream and butter also add more fat to baked potatoes, but they are food fats, full of vitamins.

Just for fun, I thought I would include my …

Basic Bread Recipe:
- 3 cups of liquid (water produces the fluffiest bread, milk and eggs a chewier texture, juice a unique flavor good for breakfast breads).[21]
- 1 Tablespoon yeast
- 1 Tablespoon salt
- 5-6 ½ cups of flour. The amount depends on the brand of flour and the humidity in the air. If you bake bread

[21] Half this recipe for a 1 ½ lb bread machine loaf. Use three cups of flour.

on a rainy day, it will take more flour than on a dry day. Flour can be white (if all white, reduce yeast by 50%) or whole wheat. You can replace up to half of the wheat flour with another type of flour; bean, oat, rice, etc.

Optional:

2± Tablespoon fat (butter or olive oil) makes the texture firmer and easier to cut.

2± Tablespoon sweet (honey, molasses, maple syrup, applesauce) mellows the whole grain flavor for those that are not used to it and helps the yeast rise faster.

1± cup fruit, veggies, nuts, instant potatoes. Added flavor, interest and nutrition. Just fun to play with.

Mix all the ingredients except the flour together.

Add the flour a little at a time until you can't stir it with a spoon.

Turn the dough out onto a floured surface and continue kneading in flour until the dough is about the texture of Play Dough and is not sticky anymore.

Place it in a greased bowl, covered with a wet towel, in a draft free place.

Let it rise until twice its starting size (1 ½ -2 hours usually, but depends on the tempreture). Punch down and knead briefly.

Let rise again (it will take less time this time.) Punch down and shape into loaves (two) or rolls, placing them in the bread pans or in a cake pan. Let rise again.

Bake at 450 for 20 minutes. Lower temperature to 400 for an additional 20 minutes (less for rolls) until they are golden brown. Take out of the oven and rub with butter or egg white and let cool for 20 minutes. Eat.

Bread is called the staff of life. Just always remember that Jesus is the Bread of Life. We need Him more than we need healthy food. He is the only Bread that can bring true health; the health of a right place with God.

13.   *Let's Visit the Barn*

Dairy and Eggs

"If the LORD delight in us, then he will bring us into this land, and give it to us; a land which flows with milk and honey." Numbers 14:8

We have studied the orchard, vegetable garden and large crop fields. Now we are going into the barn.

I picture my barn as a big, two story, traditional, red and white farm barn. The feed for the animals is stored upstairs. The center aisle is lined with neat stalls filled with clean, healthy, happy animals. They are inside in the daytime during the summer to avoid the heat and flies; and inside during the night in the winter to stay warm and toasty.

What we will bring into the house from the barn are those animal products that can be harvested without killing the animal such as milk, eggs and wool, (except we won't eat the wool.)

Over in a corner is the milking parlor. It has a stanchion (a set of bars to hold the animal still during milking) with a feed trough on the other side. Small farmers with several cows will tell you that at milking time the animals will wait at the gate and even call the farmer to let them into the barn. When he opens the gate they will each go to their own stanchion and wait for their food, sometimes not too patiently. They enjoy the relief of being milked.

All mammals produce milk for their young. Even we humans will do this. God has designed breastmilk to be the ideal food for human babies. For thousands of years, this was the only real food available for our little ones. The human race has thrived on this early food.

The nutritional content of the milk from the mother of a new born is different than milk from the mother of a three month old. Milk in the winter is higher in fat than milk in the summer (to keep baby warm) and milk produced in the summer is higher in water; just what a baby needs in the heat. There is even a light differenc e between the milk of a mom of a boy and the mom of a girl! This is a very miraculous invention of God's.

Babies who are fed artificial breastmilk (formula) have more colds, flues, and infections, dental problems, obesity, Diabetes, and speech problems.

Mothers who choose artificial milk have more trouble losing their "baby weight," regaining tone of the uterus (nursing releases oxytocin which contracts the uterus), and usually get less rest (you have to sit down once in a while to nurse. You can't prop the breast in the baby's mouth and go back to work), have higher rates of breast cancer, and usually have a less firm bond with their babies.

Nursing encourages the female body to be viewed as something other than a plaything. Breasts are more than a sex toy!

Formula is much more expensive. It cost much less to provide mom with the extra peanut butter sandwich she needs per day in order to nurse than formula does. A can of dry formula (the cheapest form) costs upwards of $10.00 each and will last from a week (for a newborn) to a day for an older child.

Most women can nurse their babies. Sometimes they need a little help because, though nursing is the most natural skill in the world, it is still a skill. Like with all skills, you have to learn how to do it.

When everyone nursed, it was much easier to learn. Today, many young mothers have never seen a baby nursing and this causes problems. You hold a baby differently to nurse (tummy to tummy) than to bottle feed (flat on his back). Also, you aim a bottle nipple at the center of the mouth while you aim the breast at the top of the mouth.

To position a baby correctly, put their tummy on your tummy, and get the baby to open his mouth as wide as possible and put as much of the dark part of the breast (areola) into his mouth as possible (rub your nipple on his mouth. It will stimulate his instinct to open up). Make sure he doesn't tuck his lip up into his mouth while aiming for the roof of his mouth.

Go to a La Leche meeting, ask a friend to let you watch them nurse, or search the Internet for videos of women nursing.[22] If you have problems, contact a Lactation Consultant.

I do have to admit, sometimes it hurts. I have had nine babies. With two of them I had extreme pain. This turned out to be because the frenulum (the pice of skin connecting the tongue to the bottom of the mouth) was too short to allow them to latch on right. This is called being "toungue-tied." For various other reasons, this caused me to have to quit nursing my oldest at one week. But with my eigth (after sucessfully nursing her other six siblings and without the other complicating factors) I simply determened to stick it out. I only nursed in absolute, text-book perfect position, was careful about

[22] I bought an excellent one from http://www.drjacknewman.com/

hygene, and took tylonol. Within two weeks her frenulum stretched out enough the pain went away. Was it easy? NO! Was it worth it? ABSOLUTLY! She ended up nursing for fifteen months.

Engorgement and a bit of tenderness as your breasts get used to their new job are normal. Again, it's worth it to simply stick it out until you, your body and baby get the hang of it all.

Once you both do get the hang of breastfeeding, it is the original "plug and play." For several reasons, my first was a bottle baby, but the rest of my children have been breastfed, so I have both experiences to campare. Nursing is WAY easier once baby gets the hang of it. No bottles to wash or formula to mix. If baby is hungry, just plug him in.

Some women, for health reasons (such as cancer or medications that are not good for baby), cannot nurse. For those women, I am glad we have the modern formulas. They are supirior to what was available before. But if at all possible, nurse your baby. It is best for both of you.

Most women who are told they "can't" nurse their babies simply need some help to get it right. Doctors aren't given classes on breastfeeding in medical school and they don't really know how to solve any problems (how can you know what you haven't been taught?) If you have a problem, get in touch with your local Le Leche League leader[23]. She is trained to help with problems in breast feeding and can direct you to more help if you need it.

[23] http://www.lll.org/

You can know your baby is getting plenty if he is peeing (six or more times a day) and pooping (at least once) and gaining weight. If he isn't, make a point of nursing more often. Milk production functions on a supply-and-demand basis. Nursing more makes your body produce more milk. This will give baby what he needs.

Mommy truly not having enough milk is such a rare event that it is not likely to happen, though many physicians will blame mommy and tell her to supplement if there is any problems at all. He simply hasn't been taught different. Contact LaLeche League if you have any problems before you give up or even choose to supplement.

Remember, too, it is normal for a baby to loose weight after birth. The IV most women have during labor sends a large amount of water to Baby as well as Mommy, making baby look like he weighs a lot more than he does (we all know what water retention does to any scale!) The first few days, he will pee all that extra out, losing several ounces of weight. This is not a sign of low milk supply, but a sign of the human body balancing itself out. If baby is peeing and pooping, he is getting plenty of milk. If it is coming out, it must be going in.

Cow's milk

…was, of course, made for baby cows and goat's milk was made for baby goats. This does not, however, mean that humans should not drink them.

I have heard it said that no other animal drinks milk after weaning. This is not exactly true.

The only thing that keeps most animals from continuing to drink milk is that they either get too big to reach the "spigot" or mama decides she is tired of feeding them and chases them away any time they try to nurse.

On farms it is common for the spring pig to be raised almost entirely on the left over milk produced by the cow right after she calves (This is when production is the highest- often 5-10 gallons per day; far more than any normal family can use even with feeding a calf, too.) Dogs, cats, goats and even chickens and horses will all enjoy a good measure of milk added to their feed and benefit from it. God created the cow to produce enough milk to feed twins, in case she should ever have them. But twins are about as rare in cows as they are in humans, so your average cow easily gives far more milk than needed just by her calf.

Of course modern breeding methods have increased that amount even more.

I heard of one man who bought four dairy cows and sixteen, day-old calves. Each of those big, black and white beauties nursed all four of her adopted calves with no problem!

Goat milk is sometimes easier to digest. Its fat and protein structure are closer to that of human milk.

"Whole milk" is 3.25% fat, 3% protein, 5% lactose sugar, and 87% water, plus many vitamins and minerals.[24] Gram for gram, it is often the cheapest form of protein available (and next to oxygen and water, protein is the most essential nutrient there is. You will die sooner without protein than any other nutrient).

---

[24] "Drink This, Not That" by David Zinczenko. I highly recommend the entire "Eat This, Not That" series. It is packed full of nutritional information and does the foot work of comparing different products to find the healthiest for you.

It also is high in many vitamins and minerals. Calcium is the most abundant. Two cups of milk (16 ounces) per day will give you your recommended amount of this bone building mineral (as will four cups of raw spinach or other dark green leafy vegetable).

Milk drinkers have less colon cancer than non-milk drinkers.

One ounce of cheese or eight ounces of yogurt are the same, nutritionally, as one cup of milk. Low fat varieties upset the natural fat/protein ratio God put in there in the first place, making it harder for your body to use the protein in the milk. Children, especially, need the high fat kind, or they need you to use real butter to cook with, or both. Fat is what the body uses to create neural pathways. Their brains will not develop right without it.

In fact, you should use real butter anyway. Margarine was not originally created as a health food, but as a cheap alternative to butter. It is made up of hydrogenated vegetable fats. These are the things that clog your arteries. (See the chapter 15 "Fat of the Land")

I once read about a study done with pigs (their digestive systems are very close to ours). One group of pigs was fed nothing but butter and the other was fed margarine. When both groups were butchered, the butter pigs had pristine arteries. Perfectly clean. The margarine pigs already had the beginnings of heart disease. The study was only six weeks long! Imagine what their arteries would have looked like after twenty years!

Another study had some men who had had heart attacks eat butter as their only fat and others ate margarine. The butter ones had far fewer repeat attacks.

In other words, God made the butter. Man made the margarine. Who do you trust to make the healthier product?

For those that are curious, butter is made by letting the natural cream in the milk rise to the top, skimming it off and shaking or stirring it until it congeals into butter[25]. The butter milk (liquid left over in the jar or churn) is rinsed out, the butter washed and salted and molded into what ever shape you want it to be (sticks, in our country, though, old time farmers wives would often mold it into many different decorative shapes). It is then ready to serve. Less processing than is needed to turn wheat into bread.

Our modern dairy products are fortified with extra vitamin D. You need D in order to use the calcium you take in. Your body makes D when your skin is exposed to sunlight. At the turn of the century, many minority children (dark skin is less efficient at absorbing sunlight), living in the shadows of the tall skyscrapers with air pollution, and wrapped up against the cold simply didn't absorb enough sunlight. By adding D to their milk the government stopped the rise of Rickets (vitamin D deficiency disease.)

Today, Rickets is again on the rise. Children are spending all their time indoors at the TV and computer, slather on sunscreen if they do go out, and parents are feeding them sodas instead of milk either because it is cheaper or in a misguided effert to avoid fat. Rickets causes the bones to grow crooked and weak. Definitely something to be avoided.

---

[25] Little Miss Muffet's "Curds and Whey" was what we call cottage cheese. The English call it "Bubble and Squeak."

What is the difference between "raw milk" and what we buy in the store?

Milk you buy in the store has been pasteurized, homogenized and fortified with vitamins D_2 and D_3.

"Pasteurization" is heating a food product to a high temperature in order to kill all the bacteria. The problem is it destroys the good bacteria and lactic acid (which helps you digest your food and fights bad bacteria) as well. This leaves a very small amount of bad bacteria with no competition for food, allowing it to multiply.

Pasteurization was begun eighty years ago because dairy cows near cities were fed the leftovers from distilleries and city garbage. 65% of these cows had Tuberculoses. They were kept on filthy feed lots and milked under unsanitary conditions. I wouldn't drink unpasteurized milk produced under these conditions either.

Today's dairies milk under much more sanitary conditions and all cows are tested once per year for tuberculoses. Any cow testing positive is immediately destroyed.

Certified Raw milk (only available in a few states) is inspected on a daily basis (far more often than normal dairies and the facilities must be almost surgically clean) and tested for pathogens. Bacteria numbers must be lower (10,000 parts per cubic centimeter) even than post-pasteurized milk (25,000 parts per cubic centimeter). Also, Certified Raw milk is often from cows who actually live on pasture instead of feed lots. This is the difference in sanitation between a pigpen and a golf course.

Pasteurization also:

- Destroys at least 90% of digestive enzymes- especially lactase- leaving anyone who doesn't produce their own, dairy intolerant. (The test to make sure pasteurization is successful is to see that there are no digestive enzymes detectable in the milk.) Digestive enzymes are what help the body assimilate all nutrients.
- Destroys amino acids lysine and tyrosine which makes proteins less available.
- Destroys many vitamins including 50% of C, 80% of the B's, 2/3 of A and D, all of vitamin B_{12},
- Destroys 50% of the minerals, including calcium. This destruction of calcium leaves pasteurized milk consumers more susceptible to osteoporosis. It also destroys chloride, magnesium, phosphorus, potassium, sodium and sulphur as well as many trace minerals.
- Destroys the Wulzen factor related to the prevention and treatment of arthritis.
- Alters the protein making it easier to be allergic.
- Alters the lactose (literally "milk sugar") making it more absorbable. This not only adds unneeded sugar to the human system, but puts stress on the pancreas leading to diabetes.
- Has been linked to chronic fatigue, and other degenerative diseases.

What is homogenization?

Homogenization is the forcing of milk through microscopic holes, which breaks up the fat molecules into much smaller pieces. This makes the fat stay thoroughly mixed in the milk instead of rising to the top like normal. This produces a prettier product that lasts longer on the store shelf.

Homogenization also:

- Causes more fat to absorb into the blood. This raises the amount of absorbable calories.
- Has been linked to increased heart disease because more fat gets into the circulatory system and thus more is able to stick to the arteries.
- May contribute to cancer. Studies have shown butter to protect against cancer, but homogenized milk does not. No studies have not yet been done on un-homogenized milk, but it would stand to reason that milk with unaltered butterfat in it would have the same results as butter. The fact is that homogenized/pasteurized fat particles go rancid faster than natural ones. Rancid fats are a known carcinogen.

What about vitamins D2 and D3?

The vitamin D that we absorb from sunlight is D_1. This is the natural kind. D_2 and D_3 are derived from toxic substances. Now, it is better to have even these types of D than nothing, but D_2 and D_3 have been linked to heart disease and are difficult to absorb.

Hormones?

Many of our dairy cows are fed hormones (Estrogen) to make them produce more milk. Feedlot beef (most of what you find in stores) is also fed Estrogen in order to make them gain weight faster. Trace amounts of hormones are found in our milk and meat. This…

- May be the cause of so many women having hormone related problems today. Some researchers say the problems are definitely symptoms of estrogen overload.[26]
- Is doing who knows what to our men!

Antibiotics?

These animals are routinely fed antibiotics, which also find their way into our food. The unnatural conditions which they are raised in cause stress, reducing their natural immunities. This reduced immunity combined with overcrowded, mucky living conditions is the perfect environment for spreading disease. Thus the routine antibiotics.

This causes common germs to become immune to antibiotics putting us all at risk of contracting antibiotic resistant strains of disease. An outbreak of salmonella in 1985 in Illinois made 14,000 people sick, killed at least one and was alarmingly genetically resistant to penicillin and tetracycline. This is likely to happen more and more often.

What else?

Chemicals to suppress odor are added (fresh-from-the-cow milk begins to smell "milky" after about two days).

---

[26] See "What Your Doctor May Not Be Telling You About Menapause/PeriMenapause" By Dr John Lee.

Powdered skim milk is added to 2% and 1% milk. The dehydration process that produces powdered milk oxidizes cholesterol making it harmful to arteries (natural, un-oxidized cholesterol is what makes our cell walls stiff and is necessary to life.) High temperature drying creates compounds that are known carcinogens and glutamic acid which is toxic to the nervous system.

Add to all this the unnatural, high protein diet the cows are fed (in order to increase production). This high protein (soybean and corn) diet has been linked to altered proteins in milk that cause milk allergies and diabetes.

Organic Milk

…Costs a little more, but for normal sized families, not enough to make a big difference in the budget (my family, however would spend at least an additional $360 a year!) Organic milk has "75% more Beta-carotene,70% more omega-3 fatty acids, 50% more vitamin E, two to three times the antioxidants lutein and zeaxanthin."[27] Organic fed cows don't receive the antibiotics or growth hormones that "normal" cows get.

Raw Milk

…has all the things God originally put into milk. It is the most complete of all foods. There is no place in the Bible that calls milk or any milk product anything but a blessing.

---

[27] "Drink This, Not That" by David Zinczenko. I highly recommend the entire "Eat This, Not That" series. It is packed full of nutritional information and does the foot work of comparing different products to find the healthiest for you.

When you buy a bottle of raw milk, you will see a layer of cream-colored liquid at the top. This is real cream. You can shake it back into the milk, skim it off and use it as cream (in your coffee or ?), whip it with a little sugar or honey for whipped cream, or keep going and it makes butter.

The milk itself can be drunk, made into buttermilk, yogurt, kefir, or many different cheeses (all with or without the cream still in it).

Unfortunately, raw milk is illegal to sell for human consumption in most states. If you look carefully you may be able to find someone willing to sell it to you illegally (raw milk is the second most common black market item, after illegal drugs, in America), though I don't really recommend breaking the law. Instead, contact your state officials and make a case for changing the laws so you have options. Or just buy your own cow or goat.

Milk is an issue everyone needs to research and decide for themselves. I do believe raw and organic (no estrogen, no antibiotics) is better if you can afford it. But the benefits of pasteurized, homogenized, hormone-ized milk are still worth having. My children and I are all milk drinkers and enjoy store bought milk when we don't own a cow, though we prefer the cow.

Low Fat or Whole?

Studies have shown that milk drinkers have an easier time maintaining their weight than none milk drinkers and the amount of fat doesn't make a lot of difference. Nor does the level of fat appear to affect your blood cholesterol. Some research sugests that milkfat helps milk protein digest and be ussed by the body better, but we're not sure yet. So drink whichever tastes best to you.

How about artificial milks?

I know more about these than I ever wanted to. When my eighth child was a week old, she began to show definite colic signs. A little experimenting told me that whenever I had milk, she had a tummy ache. Cheese, yogurt and even butter had the same (though less severe) effect. So I didn't eat pizza or any other dairy for six months, at which point she showed much more tolerance as long as I didn't go nuts. By the time she was two and a half, she could eat ice cream, yogurt, cheese and butter without much if any problem. But a glass of the liquid stuff made her sick (green/gray frothy runs with tummy aches).[28] She got her own special "milk." Raw wasn't nearly as bad, but is illegal to sell in our state, so was not an option until we can got another cow. Goat was the same as cow for our Jane, but some dairy intolerants can drink goat when they can't cow.

Lactose free milk has the digestive enzymes added to it that lactose intolerant people are lacking. If you are allergic to milk sugar (lactose) these milks are great. Unfortunately, our Jane was allergic to the protein in milk, so, though she did better on the lactose free, she was still sick.

Soy milk is made from ground up soy beans. Soy beans are high in phyto-estrogens and may very well

[28] By the time she was three and a half, she appeared to be over any allergies. Today at five she loves normal store-bought milk.

mess up men's fertility and increase a woman's risk of cancer. If, however, a woman has had a hysterectomy, she may find relief from symptoms of menopause by drinking soy. Many feel it is the best milk substitute out there, but my daughter didn't like the taste.

Rice is about the least nutritious of all grains, so rice milk isn't exactly the best idea running. It is high in sugars and low in protein. It is made by blending brown rice with water, straining out the solids and adding some vitamins and minerals.

Almond milk is made much the same way as rice milk (I have a book here with the recipe in it!) It is relatively low in protein compared to cow's milk, but as long as you don't get the sweetened flavors such as vanilla and chocolate (which of course my daughter prefers), it is low calorie. The manufacturers add some vitamins and minerals to make it come closer to real milk nutritionally.

Kefir is a fermented milk product much like yogurt only more liquid. It is packed full of vitamins and minerals and is great for you. Yogurt, buttermilk and kefir (all fermented milk products) are great additions to any diet since the bacteria that turns them from milk to these other products is the good bacteria in our intestines that helps us digest our food. Watch out for added sugar though. They have a tendency to have more sugar than anything else.

Yogurt is made by adding some yogurt (1 Tablespoon ish) to a quart of cooled (110 degrees or less), pasurized milk (you can home pasturize milk by heating it to 180 degrees for 2 minutes. This kills enzymes, as I said earlier, but these enzymes interfer with the bacteria in the yogurt) for a couple of hours. Let this sit in a warm place (80 degrees, plus or minus).

Kefir is supposed to be simplier, but I have never really been successful at it.

Here's a recepie for heavenly mozzarela cheese:

1 ½	teaspoon	**citric acid dissolved ½ cup water**
¼	teaspoon	**liquid rennet diluted in ¼ cup water**
1	gallon	**milk**

Directions:
1. Pasteurize milk.
2. Cool to 100.
3. Add acid and rennet stirring constantly.
4. Set for 5-10 minutes.
5. Cut.
6. Heat to 105-110 while stirring for 5 minutes.
7. Drain.
8. Microwave for 1 minute.
9. Knead.
10. Microwave for 30 seconds x 2, kneading between.
11. Add 1 teaspoon salt, knead and shape.

I have no idea how well this recepie keeps, since it never lasts long enough to even cool in our house.

What about cheese?

Real cheese is high in protein and calcium. The extra calcium may help strengthen you teeth when you chew it.

Cheese is made by allowing or encouraging milk to clabber, adding rennet (generally made from the lining of the stomach of young calf though there are vegetarian varieties), and allowing the mixture to age. Then the curds (solids) are cooked and drained (the whey often being fed to livestock though I understand it can be made into a lovely lemon ade like drink), pressed into a mold and aged some more. The harder the cheese the longer the processing. Cottage cheese is made by stopping after the cooking while all hard cheeses (i.e. cheddar) must be aged six months or more by law. Low fat varieties are available though nasty tasting. It takes about a gallon of milk to make a pound of cheese.

Cheese food, Velveeta, American cheese,[29] and cheese whiz are not exactly cheeses. They have some real cheese in them but often also have added fats and sugars. Not exactly good for you.

Egg-sighting!

Hens produce eggs as part of their natural reproductive cycle. They produce them whether they ever see a rooster in their life or not. The eggs you buy in the store are infertile unless marked otherwise. They would never hatch into a chick no matter how long you sat on them (the little white string you sometimes see is a ligament that holds the yolk centered).

The white of an egg is high in protein and the yolk is high in protein, vitamins and minerals; about four grams of protein total with 57 calories, and;

- 2% of your calcium,
- 4% of your vitamin A,
- 9% of your Riboflavin and
- 3% of your iron.

---

[29] Kraft brand American Cheese has far more real milk than other brands. It's almost real cheese.

Eggs are, in fact, your highest natural source of lecithin, the heart-disease fighting chemical. I have read of some doctors that actually advise you eat at least one egg per day! Let me say that again...

Eggs Are Good For Your Heart!

The studies that said otherwise used dehydrated egg yokes. That would be sort of like saying "Vodka will make you drunk so you should never eat potatoes." This simply makes no sense.

God-made potatoes are good for you. Man made (from potatoes) Vodka is bad.

God-made eggs are good for you. Man made dehydrated egg yokes are bad.

Jesus said,

"If your son shall ask for an egg will you give him a scorpion?... If you then, being evil, know how to give good gifts (eggs!) **unto your children: how much more shall your heavenly Father give the Holy Spirit to them that ask Him?"** Luke 11:12

Artificial eggs are made from egg whites, sugar, salt, and food coloring. Does that sound like good stuff to you?

Think of the good things you want to give your children. God wants to give you even better things. We think about toys. He thinks about Heaven.

But you can refuse a gift. If you try to buy something for your child and they say "No thank you," will you force them to take it? Not usually (though I do know of one woman who threatened to spank her child to get him to taste M&M's. He thought they were medicine!) God won't force His gift of salvation on you either. He offers it. Frequently. The Bible says:

"Behold, I stand at the door, and knock: if any man hear my voice, and open the door, I will come in to him, and will sup with him, and he with me." Revelation 3:20

He is standing at your heart's door right now asking to come in; asking to give you the very special gift of salvation, free room and board in the **"Land flowing with milk and honey."** All you have to do is accept it.

14.   *The Meat of the Matter*

Dead Animals and the Cross

"Look! The Lamb of God, who takes away the sin of the world!" John 1:29

The last place on our farm to explore is our pasture. It has lots of grass and some flowers here and there. A few shade trees dot the land. Contented young animals graze here; calves, lambs, goat kids, even a deer or two that have jumped the fence to enjoy the bounty. There are a few chickens pecking around (a breed raised just for meat, unlike the egg layers in the barn.) Our pasture is the place for growing up animals to eat.

This chapter is being written in the Christmas season. I thought this very appropriate. You see, our eating of meat is the object lesson for Jesus' sacrifice. In order for us to eat a steak, pork chop or drumstick an animal must give its life. They die in order to nourish our bodies. Jesus died in order to nourish our souls.

The animal's sacrifice means we have some of the essential nutrients that we need in order to live. Jesus' sacrifice means we have everything we need in order to live forever.

Today, many subscribe to the New Age, animal rights ideas; "A boy is a dog is a rat is a flea." This is an actual quote from one of the leaders of the animal rights movement. In other words, killing that flea that is nibbling on your arm is the same thing as killing your own child. They have turned things upside down; Those who kill animals are evil while those who don't are "saved." The elevating of animals to the level of humans lowers humans to the level of animals. Why would it be wrong for the government to do tests on you without your knowledge or against your will? Because you are MORE than an animal!

What did God do when Adam and Eve sinned by eating the fruit He had forbidden them? He killed a sheep and covered them with the skin. The sheep's sacrifice covered their wrong doing for a while. But it eventually wore out and had to be replaced. Jesus' sacrifice will never wear out. It will never have to be replaced.

God commanded Moses to have the children of Israel sacrifice sheep, goats and cows for every sin. This was to "pay the rent on sin," as it were.

"For it is not possible that the blood of bulls and of goats should take away sins." Hebrews 10:4

Blood sacrifices can't take away sins, only postpone the payment. (Read the whole chapter in Hebrews to get the complete message.)

Why does there have to be this sacrifice?

"For all have sinned, and come short of the glory of God;" Romans 3:23

Sin is the natural state of humanity. We are all born to sin. It is in our genetic coding. We inherited it from our Father Adam.

Babies are not held accountable for their sin. The Bible says that God does not punish us for our parent's sins and **"Therefore to him that knows to do good, and does it not, to him it is sin."** James 4:17. A child too young to know to do good can not sin. I believe babies and toddlers that die go to heaven. God is a just God and there are many examples in the Bible that support this idea.

However, no one else has an excuse. We know better but still choose to sin. No one is dragged into sin. We all run to it freely. It feels good and right and even natural to us.

"For the wages of sin is death;" Romans 6:23

Every time you sin, even a "harmless little white lie," you have condemned yourself to hell – eternal death. But this verse goes on...

"but the gift of God is eternal life through Jesus Christ our Lord."

You sinned, incurring the debt of sin. In the Old Testament, they sacrificed the animals in order to hold off the carrying out of that sentence, but a new sacrifice had to be made every year. A mere animal wasn't sufficient enough to make full payment. Jesus (the only sinless person to ever walk this planet, the only one who was not under the condemnation of death and did not deserve to die) gave Himself as the ultimate sacrifice to pay our debt of sin. It was a gift from Him to us.

"And he took bread, and gave thanks, and broke it, and gave unto them, saying, 'This is my body which is given for you: this do in remembrance of me.'" Luke 22:19

Jesus' body was broken for our sins, just as that bread was broken in His hand that day; just as that animal's body is broken for your supper. Every time we eat, we are to remember what Jesus did for us. Eating animals is one way to keep this foremost in our mind.

It was certainly easier in the days when we had to kill our own food to remember this. When we had to go out and take the life of that 1000 pound calf being butchered that we watched being born and even fed from a bottle, it really drove the seriousness of sacrifice home. Today with our sanitized meat counters in our grocery stores, we are so far removed from this concept of sacrifice that it makes it easier to not remember Christ as often as He commanded us to.

Now for the health aspects.

In the beginning, God gave all the plants to all the animals as food. There were no meat eaters. (Genesis 1:29-31)

It was only after the flood that God gave permission for humans to eat meat. Some Creation Scientists believe there was some essential nutrient in the soil that was destroyed or washed away during the flood and that nutrient can now only be attained through animal flesh. What we already know:

Vitamin B_{12} is available only in tiny amounts in plants (so tiny it is impossible to get enough from plant sources and what you get isn't metabolized right anyway), but abundant in animal products, especially meat. B_{12} is used by the body to make the nerves in the brain. Not enough B_{12}? Neurological and brain damage is very possible, especially to the children born to vegetarian mothers.

Vitamin B_3 - Niacin- available in animal products. A mild deficiency of vitamin B_3 (or niacin) may result in

A Coated Tongue	Nervousness	Insomnia
Sores In The Mouth	Skin Lesions	Chronic Headaches
Irritability	Diarrhea	
	Forgetfulness	

Digestive   Disorders   Anemia

Severe prolonged deficiency may cause neurasthenia (weakness of the nerves), mental disturbances, depression, mental dullness, and disorientation.

Iron- Iron is an essential component of hemoglobin, the oxygen-carrying pigment in the blood. Iron is normally obtained through the food in your diet and by recycling iron from old red blood cells. Without it, the blood cannot carry oxygen effectively -- and oxygen is needed for the normal functioning of every cell in the body. Symptoms of deficiency;

Pale skin color
Fatigue
Irritability
Weakness
Shortness of breath
Sore tongue
Brittle nails

Unusual food cravings (called pica)
Decreased appetite (especially in children)
Headache
Blue tinge to sclera (whites of eyes)

Note: There may be no symptoms if anemia is mild.

Essential Amino Acids- those amino acids our bodies do not make for themselves. Amino acids are the building blocks of protein which is what muscle is made of. Without the right ones we are going to suffer from severe problems. All animal proteins (milk, eggs, meat) have all the essential amino acids. No plant product does (though soybeans come close). Now, you can make a plant dish into a "complete protein" (has all the amino acids) by combining legumes with grains. But a steak does the same thing. (For more information on vitamins and minerals see the appendix).

By the time of Moses, God commanded Israel to eat red meat (lamb or kid) at least once per year. You were kicked out of the country if you didn't. Now, the main reason for this was spiritual. They needed to pay the rent on their sins. But I believe God chose to have them eat the sacrifice and not just burn it up because He knew they needed the vitamins and minerals in the meat. He, in fact, told them they could eat all the clean meats they wanted to.

"When the LORD thy God shall enlarge thy border, as he has promised thee, and thou shalt say, I will eat meat, because thy soul longs to eat meat, thou may eat meat, whatever thy soul LUSTS after." (emphasis mine) Deuteronomy 12:20 See also Deuteronomy 12:15, and Deuteronomy 12:21

Let's follow the logic;

God loves Israel.

God knows everything.

God knows whether eating red meat causes heart disease and cancer or not (as some in our culture think).

God told Israel they HAD to eat it at least once per year and were allowed to eat it as often as they wished.

Fallible, human doctors (who revise their opinions every few years) say red meat is bad.

Hmmm. I think I will take God's word for it that it is good.

To be honest, fish and fowl were the only meats most Israelites could have afforded to eat every day. You have to have a family that would make mine look tiny to eat a whole cow every other day (God told them to not eat meat that was more than two days past butchering). If you lived in the city, you could probably get fresh beef everyday and anyone could eat sheep if they had some neighbors over or butchered the animal while it was still small. But red meat would still have been a treat. Maybe a frequent one, but still a treat.

I believe we should not worry too much about the amounts of red meat we eat, though. I do believe we should try to make that meat as healthy as we can afford.

Growers put hormones (Estrogen) into their animals to get them to grow faster. They also routinely give them antibiotics to prevent the spread of disease. If you can afford it, buy Certified Organic and grass fed meat to avoid these additives. There is a possibility that the increase in "female problems" in the past century are due to these hormones and the antibiotic-resistant bacteria beginning to show up in our society are due to excessive amounts of antibiotics in our lives. The amounts that actually make it into the meat are so small that it *probably* has no affect on us, but if you can afford to avoid it, why take chances?

Actually, ideally, you would grow your own meat. Then you would know what went into the animal (Mad Cow Disease is possibly linked to feeding meat to cattle, who are supposed to be vegetarians) and could make sure it had the most pleasant life possible, with the most painless, fearless butchering possible. This, however, is not possible for most of us. Do know that I have researched this and the animals are made as comfortable as possible when dealing with the volume our big factory farms must deal with (contented cows produce more and better tasting meat on less feed than stressed, hurt, uncomfortable cows, so it is in the farmers best interest to make his cows happy). But home grown is still better.

What about those clean and unclean meats the Bible talks about? Clean meat comes from animals that chew the cud and have a split hoof, are not predatory birds (such as eagles), or that have scales and fins. This is a little harder for us at the meat counter to know the difference because we can't look at the original animal.

Beef	Duck	White fish (often
Sheep	Goose	used as artficial
Goat	Pigeon	crab meat)
Deer	Quail	Bass
Antelope	Trout	Roughy
Chicken		Tuna

are samples of clean meats.

Pork	Horse	Shark
Rabbit	Vulture	Crab
Bear	Hawk	Lobster
Camel	Catfish	

are examples of unclean meats.

In ancient Israel, you were kicked out of the country for eating the unclean meats. Eating them today will not cost you one thing as far as salvation goes. God cares about what is in your heart, not your stomach.

"Not that which goes into the mouth defils a man, but that which comes out of the mouth, this defils a man." Matthew 15:11

Jesus said your food can't send you to hell. Your speech and thoughts can.

However, there have been some studies (done by non-religious people) that have shown those meats the Bible calls unclean to be higher in toxins than those He called clean. There have also been suggestions that rheumatoid arthritis is linked to the eating of pork. There are no conclusive results yet, so use your own judgment. I, for one, still enjoy an occasional pork chop or bacon, lettuce and tomato sandwich, but it might be wiser if I didn't.

Eating unclean meat won't keep you out of Heaven. It just might get you there sooner!

Cold cuts (bologna, salami, wieners, etc.) are made by grinding meat, adding fillers (in most brands) that are basically flour and sugar, and cooking it to death. You can make these items at home, but it is a very long processes (hours of cooking at low heat). Of course, the homemade versions wouldn't have to have the sugars, fats, and preservatives that the store bought have. Basically, cold cuts and lunch meat should be kept to a minimum. There are so many additives that just aren't good for you that they outweigh most of the benefits of the meat.

You need protein at least once per day. Three times would be better as protein helps keep your blood sugar even and can be used by the body as either a carb (body energy) or a fat (brain energy). A serving of protein is the size of your palm.

And the final word?

"Look! The Lamb of God, who takes away the sin of the world!" John 1:19

15. The Fat of the Land

Good and Bad Fats

"And take your father and your households, and come unto me: and I will give you the good of the land of Egypt, and you shall eat the fat of the land." Genesis 45:18.

What is fat and is it bad for you or not? Many of us have asked this question of late. We hear many conflicting statements. Here is what I have concluded;

God made fat just the same as He made carbs and protein. He at no time forbids His people to eat all fats even when giving them health laws to live by; just the fat between the skin and the muscle (called "cover fat") and what surrounds the organs. These fats are storage places for toxins. Marbling fat inside the meat was ok.

We can grow butter and olive oil on our farm. Other fats range from "difficult to grow at home" to "impossible without a big factory."

"Fat" is a generic term for a class of lipids. Fats won't dissolve in water and have a density significantly below that of water, (they float.) Fats that are liquid at room temperature are referred to as "oil."

There are three types of fat: saturated, monounsaturated and polyunsaturated.

Saturated fats are usually solid or almost solid at room temperature. All carbon bonds on the molecule are occupied by hydrogen atoms (thus "saturated" in hydrogen). They are stable (won't easily go rancid even when heated) and your body makes them from carbohydrates as well as using the ones you eat (i.e.

animal fats, coconut oil). They constitute at least 50% of the cell membrane, giving the cell necessary stiffness and integrity so it can function properly. They help the bones absorb calcium, protect the liver from toxins, enhance the immune system, feed the heart muscle, and protect us from harmful boogie-boos in the digestive tract.

Monounsaturated fats have one double bond in the form of two carbon atoms double-bonded to each other. They are kinked at the position of the double bond. They are relatively stable also and won't go rancid when heated. They occur mostly in olives, avocados and nuts.

Polyunsaturated fats have two or more pairs of double bonds and therefore lack four or more hydrogen atoms (thus "poly or many-unsaturated"). These are also kinked. They stay liquid even in the fridge. They are unstable and go rancid very easily. Do not heat them, even in cooking, or expose them to air or light. They are found in soy, corn, Safflower, canola and other veggie oils. Excess amounts have been shown to contribute to cancer, heart disease (artery clogs are only about 26% saturated fat. The rest is unsaturated with over half of that being polyunsaturated), immune system dysfunction, liver damage, digestive disorders, learning disabilities, impaired growth, and weight gain.

All fats have at least a little of each of these, though most have more of one (such as butter which is very high in saturated fats and very low in the other two.)

Cholesterol is a high-weight alcohol that is manufactured in the liver and most human cells. Along with saturated fats, it gives our cells necessary stiffness. It is a precursor to the sex hormones, vitamin D, and vital corticosteroids (hormones that help protect us from stress, heart disease and cancer).

Bile salts, which are vital to digestion, are made from it.

Cholesterol is an antioxidant (which is why our levels go up with age. Our cells produce more of it to fight free-radicals which cause cancer and heart disease), builds neural-pathways (babies MUST have it to build their brains), and build the stomach wall.

The body produces more cholesterol, not when you eat more cholesterol, but when there are potential disease-causing conditions in your body; much like a city with a high crime rate often has a bigger police force. You don't lower the crime rate by firing your policemen, right? You don't lower your cholesterol rate by not eating cholesterol.

What causes these disease conditions? Free-radicals (cancer causers), poor thyroid function (often caused by high sugar and low vitamin and low usable iodine consumption, though there may also be a viral component), rancid fats (the ones listed above that spoil quickly and shouldn't be heated), mineral deficiencies, white flour, high counts of bacteria and bad microbes.

Triglycerides are a fancy name for fats in the human body.

HDL and LDL, the so-called "good" and "bad" cholesterols.

HDL is called good because it is higher in people who are healthy with no signs of heart disease. LDL is higher in people who are ill. LDL doesn't cause heart attacks or illness, but is a sign that there is illness in the body. High HDL is a sign of health, especially a sign of someone who exercises enough. If your LDLs are too high it means you are not exercising enough or eating good enough to keep disease at bay, or that something else has gone wrong with your body.

Hydrogenated fats are created by turning polyunsaturates (liquid oils) into solids (margarine, shortening). To do this manufacturers start with the cheapest oils (soy, corn, cottonseed, etc.) which are already rancid (the oxygen and heat they are exposed to during extraction often turns them rancid from the get go). They mix them with tiny metal particles (usually nickel oxide) and subject them to hydrogen gas in a high-pressure, high-temperature reactor. Then they add soap-like emulsifiers and starch to give it a better consistency. Then the oil is steam cleaned (high-temperatures again). This removes the nasty odor. They bleach its gray color into white, dye it yellow, and add flavoring to make it resemble butter. Now doesn't that sound yummy?

Trans fats are polyunsaturated fats where, because of the chemical changes in the hydrogenation process, the hydrogen atoms change position on the fatty acid chain. Before "margarine," pairs of hydrogen atoms occur together causing the chain to bend. After hydrogenation, the atoms are on the opposite sides of the fatty chain causing the chain to straighten out. This "trans" formation is rarely found in nature. Your digestive system does not recognize these as the poisons they are. It incorporates Trans-fats into the cell membranes as though they were normal fats. Once in place they prevent necessary chemical reactions because the electrons in your cell membranes are in the wrong places so the chemicals your body needs don't fit where they belong. The spots are occupied by the useless trans-fats.

What I have just said is completely opposite of what you constantly hear in the media, isn't it? It looks like saturated fats and cholesterol are GOOD for you while polyunsaturated fats are BAD. Here is the first key; God made most saturated fats. Man made most polyunsaturated fats.

"There is a way which seems right unto a man, but the end thereof are the ways of death." Proverbs 14:12

Before 1920, when our diet consisted of 50% saturated fats, coronary heart disease was so rare, doctors advised the man importing the first electrocardiograph to go into a more profitable field.

The Framingham Heart Study of over forty years with 6,000 people found that the more saturated fat one ate, the more cholesterol one ate, the more calories one ate, and the more active one was, the LOWER the person's serum cholesterol. Now, if they were overweight and inactive, they did have a slightly higher risk of heart disease. Gee, it looks like it is TV and labor saving devices such as cars that are causing heart disease instead of butter!

A British study with several thousand men was split into two groups. Half ate less saturated fats and cholesterol and stopped smoking. The other group didn't. At the end of one year those on the "good" diet had MORE deaths than those on the "bad" diet even though the "bad dieters" kept smoking (something we know for a fact will shorten your life).

A study of 12,000 men showed that those with "good" dietary habits had a slight reduction in coronary heart disease but they were VERY much more likely to die from cancer, brain hemorrhage, suicide, and violent death, more than making up for the reduction in heart disease.

A medical research council survey showed that men eating butter ran half the risk of developing heart disease than those that used margarine.

Jews in Yemen, whose diets contained fats solely of animal origin, had little heart disease or Diabetes compared to a group of Jews living in Israel. (First clue:) The Jews in Israel ate sugar. Those in Yemen didn't.

The Masai African tribes subsist largely on milk, blood and beef. They have no heart disease and have low cholesterol.

Eskimos eat a great deal of animal fat. They have no heart disease.

In China, regions where the people consume large amounts of whole milk have half the rates of heart disease than those that consume small amounts of animal products. [30]

I could fill page after page of studies that show eating God-made fats to be healthy.

Why, then, all the hype to make everyone quit eating saturated fats and cholesterol?

"We have not lost faith, but we have transferred it from God to the Medical Profession."
George Bernard Shaw

---

[30] Nourishing Traditions by Sally Fallon

Most in science have rejected God, making humans the closest thing to divine they believe in. Certainly modern human scientists are smarter than random, natural, accidents (Evolution). Thus, many have no problem accepting that creation is flawed.

A doctor in the 1950's first proposed that eating fat caused the heart to quit working. He did some studies that showed ambiguous results, at best. But since he was already so convinced that his ideas were right, he believed the studies showed that the "Diet-Heart" idea was correct and said so in his summaries. Other scientists soon did more studies with the same idea in mind. Most of these were either so poorly done and biased as to be of no use whatsoever or else the study showed no correlation between heart disease, high cholesterol, and fat intake, but the scientists wrote in their summaries that they HAD seen a correlation.

As the years went by and the studies became bigger and more important, scientists became aware that if they didn't support the diet-heart idea they would become a laughing stock and not be able to get any more government money for research; they would be unemployed. So they would say they had found evidence that high fat/cholesterol caused heart disease whether they did or not. (Does this begin to sound like the old story "The Emperor Has No Clothes" to you?)

Most doctors are neither research scientists nor statisticians.[31] They would have a great deal of trouble reading the actual reports. That is not their specialty. Nor

---

[31] For a book on this subject written by a doctor who also happens to be a research scientist AND a statistician see "The Cholesterol Myth" by Dr. Uffe Ravnskov, MD, PhD

do they have the time to read the many pages of technical information in each report. So they do what everyone else does; they read the study director's summary of the results of the report. If the director is biased or out right lying, the doctor would have no way of knowing this anymore than we do. When the media wants to report on medical issues, they read the study summaries and talk to the doctors that read the summaries as well as the directors that wrote the summaries. Since the whole diet-heart idea sounds logical, we all try to follow the government guidelines that were set by the scientists that did the studies and the manufacturers of the cholesterol lowering drugs.

Many in the media are vegetarians for religious reasons, so anything that discredits eating animals is assumed to be right and anything that supports eating animals is wrong. Thus they ignore any studies that don't support their viewpoint (Not intentionally. There isn't enough time or money to report every little thing in the world and they have to choose to leave something out. When a study comes along that, according to your world view, can not possibly be right, you leave it off in favor of news that you see as correct).

Sugar has far more convincing links to heart disease, but the Sugar Public Relation Experts are very active in encouraging the media and doctors to ignore any evidence that may harm their product's sale. There is no "Fat Public Relations" group.

One man who is a doctor, research scientist AND statistician[32] put all the studies he could find together and read them (the whole studies, not just the summaries).

---

[32] "The Cholesterol Myth" by Uffe Ravnskov, MD, PhD

His conclusion is that there is no proof that what you eat will affect your cholesterol levels or your chance of heart disease. Nor will your cholesterol levels affect your risk of heart disease (women with high cholesterol live longer than any other group, for example.)

If you want to lower your risk of heart attack;

- Reduce the stress in your life. It has been proven that stress causes your blood vessels to restrict, reducing the flow of blood and, if there are any blockages, causing heart attacks.

The fact is that we live in a very high stress society. It used to be that only men had heart attacks. Since women entered the workforce in mass, though, their rates of heart attacks have gone up to nearly the same as men.

I don't think that is what the feminists meant when they said they wanted "equality."

A hundred years ago, everyone was a farmer and in touch with God's Creation everyday (which reduces stress in and of itself). They ate natural foods (which didn't stress the digestive system). The roles in life were clearly defined, so the hubby didn't have to worry about whether the canning got done and the wifey didn't have to worry about whether the plowing got done.

No one had to stress about how they fit into society either. You just knew because you saw where you were going and how you fit in from the time you were born. Sure, your life had its problems, but not anything you hadn't seen your parents and neighbors handle. And everything slowed down to a near stop in the winter, so your body had down time to heal while you had time to spend with your family forming those bonds that reduced your stress in the hard times.

Today, you have to decide what your place in life will be (Gay? Straight? Bi? Trans? Single? Married? Co-habittating? Conservative? Liberal? Druggy? Hippie? Preppie? Surfer? Skater? Biker? Valley girl? Yup-dink? Yup-dwk? Yup-swk? Redneck? And on and on), you have to fight your way through a very unnatural, high stress environment known as "school." Then you have to work in an unnatural environment (unless you are a professional farmer or cowboy). You are bombarded with messages to buy, Buy, BUY; both sexes have to worry about outside the home issues AND inside the home issues, plus we choose to be bombarded by messages of stress and conflict (ever seen any TV show that wasn't filled with conflict of some type or another?) for "entertainment" and "relaxation"! No wonder we are keeling over in record numbers!

Remember the best ways to reduce stress? Studies have shown that believing in God reduces all stress-caused diseases. Those who attend church regularly and pray often have fewer serious illnesses and recover from those illnesses faster. I think this is God's way of rewarding the faithful. As with most of God's rewards, the physical cause is easy enough to explain. It is just less stressful to leave all your troubles to God and trust Him to take care of them than it is to believe you are your only hope.

So, go to church, read your Bible (you will find answers to most of the above questions there. You don't have to fuss about it yourself), pray, and when you find yourself worrying, consciously place those cares on His alter and walk away.

- Exercise more. Get the blood pumping through your arteries. This stretches them and keeps them limber. Think of a piece of leather; If you let it sit in one place never moving and never do anything to care for it, it will dry up and crack into pieces. If you rub it with lubricant (a fat, by the way) and move it around and use it, it will stay supple and soft, sometimes for decades. Your arteries are the same way. Exercise makes the blood pump faster and harder which stretches the artery walls. This keeps them soft and supple. I mentioned the Masai tribe above who live on blood, beef, and milk. They also run and walk many miles everyday looking for forage for their cattle. They have NO heart disease.
- Eat naturally. Give your body the vitamins and minerals it needs to function correctly and it reduces the stress it takes to live. It also gives your body the tools it needs to repair itself.
- Avoid man-made sugars (table-sugar), and polyunsaturated fats, especially hydrogenated ones such as margarine. These substances steal from your body instead of giving to it and act as poisons.
- Enjoy your red meats and butter. God made them. Leaving them out will NOT lower your risk of heart attack. It might raise your stress level.

"The farther science strays from God, the more they will believe taboo and superstition."

You would think if eating butter and eggs and other high fat items was bad for us, God would have told us so when He told us to wash after handling diseased bodies, not to go to the bathroom in the middle of the street, and the many other sensible health laws He gave us in Deuteronomy. But there is only one statement in the Bible saying anything bad about eggs. That is in Job where he says he will not eat eggs without salt because they taste gross that way (I agree!) Jesus said eggs were a good gift, remember?

"If your son shall ask an egg will you give him a scorpion?... If ye then, being evil, know how to give good gifts (eggs!) **unto your children: how much more shall your heavenly Father give the Holy Spirit to them that ask him?"** Luke 11:12

Butter is, likewise, referred to in a good or neutral sense throughout the Bible.

Eggs are your highest natural source of Lecithin.

The second highest source of Lecithin in the American diet is butter which is anti-bacterial, anti-tumoral, boosts the immune system and is choke-full of vitamins; A, D, K, E, and all their naturally occurring cofactors. You can not absorb any minerals without sufficient quantities of these vitamins in your blood.

Butter contains the Wulzen factor which prevents stiffness of joints.

It contains Arachidonic Acid, a vital component of cell membranes and precursor to prostaglandins.

It has short chain fatty acids, which do not need to be emulsified by bile salts, but are absorbed directly from the small intestine to the liver where they are converted into quick energy (instead of being stored as body fat).

Butter contains manganese, zinc, chromium and iodine.

Gee, you would think Someone smart had designed it.

Omega 6 fatty acids aid in eye function, skin strength and pregnancy but encourage inflammation. **Omega 3's** do the same things but are less encouraging to inflammation and better at boosting the immune system. They have been shown to lower triglycerides (fat in the blood), decrease heart attacks and varicose veins, reduce scaring, depression and blood pressure. They also appear to reduce the risk of cancers and improve brain function.

Omega 3s and 6s compete for the same places in cells. You definitely want as many 3s in your diet as possible. They are found in oily fish (salmon, herring, mackerel, anchovies, tuna, shark, orange roughy, mahi mahi, and sardines; pretty much anything that has fins and scales), flax seeds, chia seed, kiwi fruit, walnuts, brown algae, black raspberry and hemp. Plant sources are not as good as the fish sources but are better than nothing. Eggs from chickens fed greens and insects (a much more natural diet than the corn and soybeans fed to most factory farm chickens) are also high in the omega 3s. The same goes for the chicken meat as well as beef, lamb and grass fed milk products. The more natural, grass fed diets produce the healthier omega 3s.

- So, eat fish at least once a week (though there is some concern about mercury poisoning in some fish. Most nutritionists believe the benefits of the omega 3s outweigh the risks of the mercury) and if you can afford, it eat range/grass fed meat, milk and eggs.

God created this world. He provided food for us. He loves us. I believe He provided the best food possible in terms of taste and health. If margarine and artificial eggs are better for us why didn't He make cows and chickens give them instead? If red meat is bad for us why didn't He tell Israel they couldn't eat it instead of saying they could have all they wanted as long as they left off the cover fat? Why didn't He tell Israel to let the cream rise to the top and discard it before drinking the milk? Why didn't He forbid eating eggs?

What did He tell us?

"There is a way which seemeth right unto a man, but the end thereof are the ways of death." Proverbs 14:12

Summary:

When you eat fat opt for those that are closest to nature; butter, olive oil, nut oils, coconut oil, etc.

Canola is the best of the light flavored oils, so use it when the others are too strong.

Eat fish at least once per week and, if possible, eat range/grass fed eggs, meat and milk.

Enjoy your meats but cut off the layer of fat around the edge. Sadly, this means the chicken skin, too.

16.   *The Salt of the Earth*

Salt

"Ye are the salt of the earth:" Matthew 5:13

We can't grow salt on our farm as it is an accumulation of chemicals from the sea. Unless our farm is close enough to the sea to have very soft water, we will need to buy our salt from somewhere.

Salt's (sodium-chloride) main function in the body is to help the nervous system transmit nerve impulses from nerve cell to nerve cell. It also helps in the production of the hydrochloric acid that is produced in the stomach and dissolves the protein in your food, absorbs some minerals (such as iron), and prevents stomach infections from bacteria and other microorganisms that you take in with your food.

Salt is a known anti-bacterial. Human blood contains 0.9% salt; the same concentration as found in the saline solution commonly used to cleanse wounds in hospitals.

It also maintains the electrolyte balance inside and outside of cells. Expectant mothers are advised to get enough salt to protect their babies ("Salt to Taste") from electrolyte imbalance and bacteria.

Increased salt intakes have been used successfully to treat Chronic Fatigue Syndrome and the unique microclimate of salt mines is a popular way to treat asthma. You would, in fact, die if you did not take in enough salt.

Americans do not generally have a problem with too little salt intake, though. Most of our salt comes from foods, some from water, especially if you live near the ocean. The National Academy of Sciences recommends that Americans consume a minimum of 500 mg/day of sodium to maintain good health. Most Americans consume about 3,500 mg/day of sodium, (seven times the recommended amount); men more than women.

Processed foods are very high in salt (a preservative- remember it kills bacteria) giving the average American way more salt than he needs for maintenance every day (A can of soup for example, has three or more times the RDA of salt).

Individual needs, however, vary enormously based on genetic make-up and the way people live their lives. The kidneys generally efficiently process this "excess" sodium in healthy people, especially those who drink plenty of water. For healthy people, too high of salt intake is not a problem. Some recent studies have even shown that a low salt diet may increase the risk for heart attacks in otherwise healthy people.

When you work hard enough to sweat or stay in a hot climate long enough, you loose a lot of salt through perspiration. You should replace this loss with water in most situations. Since water has salt as well as other minerals, it does a great job of replacing your losses. That is what God designed it for.

If you exercise like a marathon runner, an Olympic athlete, or work in a hot climate in an un-air-conditioned environment, (such as an enclosed warehouse in the south), you may need a little more than water can provide for you. That is when most people turn to sports drinks, but studies have shown that chocolate milk does a much better job of replenishing those lost minerals with fewer calories and excess salt. Wilderness hikers use salt tablets to combat hyperthermia along with plenty of water. This works great.

For 4,000 years, we have known that salt intakes can affect blood pressure through signals to the blood vessels that maintain blood pressure within a proper range. Some have suggested that since salt intakes are related to blood pressure, and since cardiovascular risks are also related to blood pressure, that salt intake levels are related to cardiovascular risk. This is the "Salt Hypothesis."

We know that a minority of the population can lower blood pressure by restricting dietary salt. Reducing blood pressure can reduce the risk of a heart attack or stroke in people with chronic high blood pressure. Blood pressure is a sign. When it goes up (or down) it indicates an underlying health concern.

Changes result from many variables, though, which are often still poorly-understood.

So if you do not have high blood pressure and are not at risk for high blood pressure don't worry too much about how much salt you eat. If you do have high blood pressure or if it runs high in your family, you are a man, smoke, or are obese (since high blood pressure has no symptoms and you won't know when you get it) you may try limiting your salt intake. Buy an inexpensive bloodpressure moniter at any drug store or Walmart and see what happens to your blood pressure when you change your diet (make sure you get an extra large cuff if you are fat since too-small a cuff will give you a false high reading) . If you see a positive response to limiting your salt intake, make some permanante changes. It will take about three months for most people's taste buds to adjust to the lower salt levels, but once they do, anything "normal" will taste nasty to you. If you don't see a difference in your blood pressure, don't worry about your salt intake.

Salt substitutes vary in their composition, but their main ingredient is always potassium-chloride with a little bit of sodium-chloride for taste. Potassium is a mineral that is found naturally in foods (bananas, orange juice, etc.) and is necessary for many normal functions of the body, especially the beating of the heart. The amounts of potassium-chloride most people get in salt substitutes are actually good for you. I seriously doubt you could possibly take enough to harm you through your salt shaker. However, don't take it intravenously in high doses. That is what a Lethal injection used by the government in executions is made from. More is NOT better.

Iodine is required as a trace element for most living organisms. In areas where there is little iodine in the diet—typically inland areas where no marine foods are eaten—iodine deficiency gives rise to goiter. Iodine deficiency is also the leading cause of preventable mental retardation. This is caused by lack of thyroid hormone in the infant. Iodine deficiency remains a serious problem that affects people around the globe. In America, this is now combated by the addition of small amounts of iodine to table salt. This product is known as "Iodized Salt." Iodine compounds have also been added to other foodstuffs, such as flour.

I know many people with under-active thyroids. This doesn't make sense when you consider that everyone in

America gets plenty of iodine in their salt. That is, it didn't make sense until I found out that fluoride (commonly added to city water to prevent cavities), bad diets (white sugar and flour, low vitamins and minerals), many of the chemicals in our foods, pesticides, alcohol, drugs and radiation from x-rays interfere with the absorption of iodine.

If you have low thyroid function, you may consider taking a seaweed or black walnut shell supplement to increase your iodine intake as well as eliminating sugar, alcohol, and other toxins from your diet and environment and adding more fruits and veggies. This just might spur your thyroid on to make more of its own hormones and reduce your reliance on synthetic thyroid medicines.

"You are the salt of the earth, but if the salt has lost his savor, wherewith shall it be salted? It is thenceforth good for nothing, but to be cast out, and to be trodden under foot of men." Matthew 5:13

Salt is necessary for life. Without it we die. It also makes life more interesting by adding flavor.

Jesus said that we are the Salt of the Earth. Without us, this world dies and has no "flavor." If we loose our "saltiness," (the light of Jesus' love shinning out of us to others), we aren't good for anything but gravel in the road, something for people to walk on. We must each make sure we have enough Jesus in our day through prayer and Bible reading to keep our "Jesus' Blood" pressure up where it needs to be. Unlike in the physical body, our spiritual body can only have too low "Blood pressure;" Never too high. Take time everyday to add some more of the Salt of God's Word to your life so you can share it with others and keep them from dying of a "heart-ache attack."

17.   *The Breath of Life*

Air Quality

My family has a history of allergies, especially those that trigger asthma.

Hubby's family has a history of allergies that trigger hives.

My kids never had a chance (though, thankfully, they appear to take more after their dad than me in this area).

So, I have done more research on allergies than I ever really wanted to.

Allergies have always been around, being recorded in ancient Greece, but their incidence is defintly increasing. In one recent article a pediatrician said ¼ of the children in his waiting room have food allergies. This doesn't even take into account the non food ones!

Though we don't really know why there is such a marked increase, and there are a lot of theories, I personally think vaccines are a major contributor, possibly with vaccine damage being passed on the cellular level to a person's children.

There has been a good deal of attention paid to outdoor air pollution, but the truth is that indoor pollution is a far more serious issue.

We spend a good deal more time inside, and pollutants build up over time, where outside they are dispersed and thinned out.

"According to the Environmental Protection Agency, the top five air quality problems in the U.S. are all indoor air problems. Common residential indoor pollutants include excessive moisture, volatile organic

compounds (VOCs), combustion products, radon, pesticides, dust particles, viruses, and bacteria. All of these are known to affect human health, and the resulting odors, dampness, stale air, and stuffiness also make a house less comfortable."
https://smarterhouse.org/ventilation-and-air-distribution/indoor-air-pollutants

How do you know if your house's air is bad?

If you have anything that burns in your house (gas stove, furnace, gas dryer, etc) there is a possibility of carbon dioxide and carbon monoxide being leaked into your house, both highly dangerous.

Mold is a serious problem, also. All molds and mildews put spores out into the air for you to breathe. Some molds are more dangerous than others, but none of them are good for you.

Animals put out dander and "dust mites." So, if you have pets, the dust level in your home will be higher, and dander and dust mites are highly allergic compounds.

If you live in the country, you likely have mice (and might in the city too). They will add to household pollution, also. As will roaches.

And humans. Most dust mites in most homes are actually shed human skin and hair.

VOC's (mentioned above) are compounds in paint, varnish, glues, dry-cleaning chemicals, markers, fire-proofing chemicals on carpets, drapes, and pajamas. Gasses dissipate into the air from any and all of these.

Let's add in that we all have electronics in our homes in some form. Electronics, pollen, dust, dirt, pollutants, and any other junk in the air carry a positive ion charge, meaning they have more protons than electrons. (If you have the same number of protons and electrons, the element is "balanced" and called an atom. If you have more electrons, we call it a negative ion, fewer electrons a positive ion.)

Since our own cells are mostly negative ions, too much exposure to the positive ones make us depressed, anxious, and fatigued. (Thunder storms, rainfall, plants, and beaches generate negative ions, explaining why we feel so much better when we go near these things. They balance us.)

It doesn't help that pesticides, household cleaners, and air fresheners all have toxic chemicals in them, also, that do damage to our bodies, especially lungs. So, you can start improving your house's air by simply not using these products any more than you have to.

The all purpose cleaner I use is:

- 1 Tablespoon of borax
- 1 Tablespoon washing soda
- 1-5 drops of dish soap (I use hypoallergenic Palmolive.)
- 1 quart of warm water
- 1 spray bottle that costs $2 or more (works better than cheap ones).

Just mix everything in the spray bottle (add the soap last so it doesn't produce too many suds). It's actually the best cleaner I've used, and it doesn't give me an asthma attack or make anyone itch. You can add a few drops of your favorite essential oil if you want. I like to use lemon, myself. Stupid-cheap as well as affective and non-allergenic.

Air fresheners don't actually freshen the air. They cover up bad odors by adding "good" oders on top, while putting positive ions into the air and pollutants into your lungs.

You can certainly hire a professional to check you air quality out for you. You can also buy some electronic detectors for your house, such as radon and carbon monoxide detectors. Amazon carries them.

Or if you have these symptoms in your family you can be pretty sure somethings wrong:

- Coughing
- Sneezing
- Watery eyes
- Nasal congestion

Or if you and your family frequently gets:

- Headaches
- Bloody noses
- Dizziness
- Nausea
- Rashes
- Fever
- Chills
- Fatigue

they may actually have allergies, not "bugs."

You're not alone.

Even if you live in a big city, odds are good the air outside is better than the air in your house, so the number one method to clean the air in your house is to open up your windows and at least get as good of quality as is outside into your house. Even as little as 5 minutes a day will make a big difference.

Now, we leave our windows open as much as possible around here, which means mid-April to somewhere in September, unless it's raining, which is seldom here since its the desert (we get about 10 inches a year). This does make a difference.

It is the high desert (4500 feet elevation), though, so for half the year it's too cold to leave the windows open very many days.This is the time of year the mold grows. Yes, its the desert, with around 20% humidity, but with all the showers, laundry, dishes, etc going on with our family of 11, we stay around 60% in the house when the windows stay closed. Much too high.

So we need to go further than opening windows.

#2 Best Way to Improve Indoor Air

Plants "breathe" in carbon dioxide and "breathe" out oxygen which makes the air feel fresher to us. They also produce negative ions for us to absorb, so we need plants around us no matter what. But it seems they also remove mold spores, pollen, dust, dander, mites, and many chemical pollutants from the air. They are living filters.

The best plants are:

- Spider plant (one of the best)
- Pothos
- Orchids (which, addition to cleaning the air, add extra oxygen into the air at night, making them great for bedrooms)
- Bamboo palm,
- Chinese evergreen,
- English ivy,
- Gerbera daisy,
- Janet Craig, Dracaena "Janet Craig"
- Marginata, Dracaena marginata
- Mass cane/Corn plant,
- Mother-in-Law's Tongue,
- Pot mum,
- Peace lily,
- Warneckii, Dracaena "Warneckii"

But, really, any plant is good.

According to NASA you need about 1 plant for every 120 square feet for optimum cleaning. So if you have the average 1200' home you need around 10 plants (with a 6-8 inch diameter pot. Bigger plants can count as more than one plant).

Do be careful not to overwater them since that will increase algae, and remove any dead leaves or stems so decaying plant matter doesn't add to the pollution in your house.

Salt Lamps

It is a known fact that people suffering with asthma get better if they go into salt mines. Breathing the salt-laden air really helps the lungs.

You can buy large lumps of salt (or baskets of small lumps) from those mines that have a light bulb in them. This is generally called "Himalayan Salt Lamps." The light gently warms the salt, causing it to absorb pollution- laden water from the air. The water then evaporates back into the air, leaving the pollutants behind. The rocks should be wiped clean a couple times a week.

The light from these "lamps" is a soft, warm orange, which mimics the sunset, encouraging sleep, so we will use ours for our night-time reading lamps.

Air filters

Charcoal will filter out many, many pollutants, and is in fact, used in most air and water filters. The most natural air filter is to just hang some activated charcoal in a breathable pouch (cheesecloth, nylon stockings) or just put some in a bowl in the rooms you want to clean. I plan to buy some soon and put some under seats in our cars, as well as throughout the house.

You could use barbeque briquettes, but they often have unhealthy additives, so read the label.

Also, activated charcoal has been treated to make it more porous, increasing the surface area to absorb pollutants, so it would be better to use than BBQ briquettes.

All charcoal would need to be replaced every couple of years.

Mechanical Air filters

I already use HEPA (High-Efficiency Particulate Air) filter bags in my vacuum cleaner to help reduce dust and yucky stuff. I try to vacuum most weekdays, which reduces the allergens in our house.

My brother has removed all carpet of any kind from his house and was able to get rid of his asthma medicines! Carpets are fuzzy dirt traps, it seems.

We will be replacing ours with hard floors of some type as they wear out. Advantage: I can install laminate flooring (helped do it in my church) so I can save installation costs by making this choice! Laminate has the problem that it is artificial and gasses out toxins into the air (as do carpets), but on the other hand, you only need plain water and a microfiber mophead to clean it, so no toxic cleaners. And mops are cheaper and last longer than vacuums do.

I was also given an air filter some years ago. It needs new filters frequently, and is only big enough to do one room- not the whole house like I need- but it will help when we must keep the windows shut.

We'll add that our house is cooled with a swamp cooler. This means all summer the air is pulled into our house through a wall of watered down pads and pushed out the open windows, filtering out many pollutants before they even come into the house.

Beeswax Candles

I have not tried these yet, but might. They release negative ions as they burn as well as cleaning pollutants out of the air.

Other Things that Will Help Allergies

Regular dusting, especially on the hard to see places like door tops, also helps. Flylady.com suggests you use a high quality feather duster that holds the dust instead of scattering it, and set a timer for 10 minutes once a week and just dust what you can in that 10 minutes. This will keep most homes pretty dust free, with the addition of just a deep dusting with a cloth once or twice a year. (and its kind of fun waving the feather duster around like a magic wand while trying to beat the timer).

Washing curtains and other "soft" surfaces, and vacuuming those you can't wash, can also drastically reduce dust and their bugaboos.

Dust-mite proof covers on all pillows and mattresses on the bed will help, also, as will washing your sheets weekly and blankets frequently. Now, I have a hard getting to this much washing, honestly. I'm not perfect. But I can do better, so I will.

Groom your pets regularly to help reduce their contributions to the atmosphere.

Keeping shoes out of the house helps too, if you can do it. I keep a large box by the door for everyone to put their shoes in. It reduces the cleaning as well as the allergens. And, at least when I had a bunch of little kids, I always had an idea where the shoes were.

Good quality doormats (such as astro turf) helps pull dirt and contamaenets off of shoes before they even get into the house. Nice big ones that people have to take a couple of steps on are best.

Natural ways to have good smelling air

If you want more scent to your air than "clean" you can bake a loaf of bread :-) or put a small pot on to simmer on the back of your stove with some cloves, vanilla beans, or any spices you enjoy the scent of. And an essential oil infuser will do a similar job.It is believed the infused essential oil will also help clean the air.

I'm not perfect. I can't do all these things. But I can do more than I do now, and will.

18.   Summary

"Beloved, I wish above all things that thou mayest prosper and be in health, even as thy soul." 3 John 1:2

We have been studying nutrition and how to be healthy. "You are what you eat" is quite true. Garbage in-garbage out as they say. Let's go over what we have studied.

- Eat five or more servings per day of fruit and veggies. (Remember a serving is what you can comfortably hold in one hand) Nine is best. This gives you the vitamins you need to function right. Your body can't do the work it needs to do without the right tools and vitamins are those tools.

I plan when I eat each; one fruit with breakfast, one veggie with lunch, a fruit snack in the evening, and one of each with supper. If I just say "I will eat more fruit." I won't do it. I have to plan it into my menu.

Now, "fruit with breakfast" can be a banana, a glass of orange juice, a handful of raisins in my cereal, or any other way I can think of. "Veggies with lunch" means carrot sticks, a side salad, or even veggie soup.

It takes a while to get in the habit of doing this, so go easy on yourself. Plan them into your menu when you shop. Prepare your fruit for breakfast the night before and do the best you can to remember it. If you do forget, though, don't kick yourself. Just do better tomorrow. It takes four to six weeks to form a new habit, so give yourself that time.

- Eat four or more servings (what you can hold in two hands or one slice of bread or a muffin) of whole grains

per day. This is getting easier and easier. More and more companies are making their products with whole grain. After all, unhealthy customers die, and dead people don't spend much money on food.
Read lots of labels. Of course, anything you can make by scratch will be healthier still.

Again, plan it in; one whole grain for breakfast, one or two for lunch, and two for supper. Remember that whole grains have vitamins, minerals and fiber just like fruits and veggies do. They are different vitamins, though, so you need both.

Ideas for whole grains: popcorn, whole wheat bread (make sure the label says 100% whole wheat or 100% whole grain), oatmeal, whole grain muffins, brown rice, raisin bran, or toasted wheat berries (grain) on your salad. Keep your eyes open and get creative.

- You need about three servings per day of protein; one for each meal. A serving of protein is the size of your palm. Your body doesn't store protein so you need to replenish it on a regular schedule. Proteins have the essential amino acids your body needs to build and maintain muscle, including your heart muscle.

I eat one serving at each meal plus an extra one in the middle of my homeschool day to keep my brain working right. Proteins are milk, cheese, yogurt, meat (beef, lamb, pork, chicken, fish, turkey, deer, rabbit, etc.) nuts, legumes (beans), or eggs (a good gift from God, remember). Soy beans are high in protein and almost all the amino acids you need, but also high in phyto-estrogens, which may contribute to hormone imbalance.

- A minimum of two servings of high calcium foods is necessary to maintain bone density. These can be dairy products (one hands- worth), dark green leafy veggies (spinach, Dandelion- two hands worth), or fish bone soup. Other ways to make sure your bones are thick enough to not break are to engage in weight-bearing exercises and don't drink sodas. Exercise adds layers to your bones and sodas remove them.

- One serving of high quality fat (such as butter or fresh nuts) is essential to your good health. You need the fat soluble vitamins from these products. Avoid man-made fats such as margarine, shortening, and hydrogenated veggie oil. These will poison your system and cause heart disease. A serving of fat is the size of your thumb, about a tablespoon.

Don't eat whites: sugar, bread, or fat. These are all highly processed and far removed from God's original design. (Cauliflower, white pumpkin, white squash, and any other white fruits and veggies don't count as "whites" despite their colors. Put them in the fruits and veggies class. And life is too short to not ever eat sweets or deserts. Your body can handle a certain amount of "Junk" and will just filter it out. The problem comes in when you overload your system so much it can't handle the junk effeciantly.)

➤ Exercise more today than you did yesterday.

Or to put all this in an easy to remember format:
5, 4, 3, 2, 1, 0, blast off.
Five-;nine servings of fruits and veggies per day.
Four+ servings of whole grains.
Three servings of protein.
Two+ servings of high calcium foods.
One serving of HIGH QUALITY fat.
Zero white things.

And **blast** that energy out of your system through exercise.

We can do more for God when we feel better and we feel better when we take care of ourselves.

Our bodies are a very special gift God has given us and we are responsible to care for them properly. Here is hoping you are all healthier.

"But my God shall supply all your need according to his riches in glory by Christ Jesus."
Philippians 4:19

Dear Readers

Be cause of on-going research in the fields of nutrition and health, I am constantly learning more about God's marvelous creation. In order to keep you updated, I have opened a blog at MrsBettyTracy.com. Please feel free to check in.

I am also on facebook. Please look me up. I would love to hear from you!

God Bless

Mrs. Betty Tracy

Appendix A- Vitamins and Minerals

Essential- In nutritional terms, "essential" means you must have it to be healthy but your body doesn't make it itself. For example, there are actually around twenty-five amino acids needed by the human body, but your body manufactures sixteen by itself. The other nine are "essential."

Human beings are one of the few animals that do not manufacture their own vitamin C; thus, to humans, vitamin C is essential while it is not to other animals.

Protein

All proteins are composed primarily of amino acids though the proportion of acids differs from one protein to another. Some can be made by the body and others (nine) are "essential"- must be supplied by the diet. You cannot digest and transport nutrients without amino acids. Unfortunately, many are destroyed by processing.

Protein is available in meat, milk, cheese, yogurt, beans, grains, nuts, and in small amounts in veggies. All protein from animals have all the essential amino acids; they are "complete." No plant sources have them all and must be combined to be complete. Generally this means combining a grain with a legume (i.e. red beans and rice, peanut butter on whole wheat bread). Many believe soy to be a complete protein. It is not, though it comes closer than other plant sources.

The essential amino acids are Isoleucine, Leucine, Lysine, Methionine, Phenylalanine, Threonine,

Tryptophan (the chemical in warm milk, and turkey that makes you sleepy on Thanksgiving), Valine,

Vitamins

Vitamins are either fat-soluble or water-soluble. That means they dissolve in either fat or water.

Water-soluble vitamins are not stored well by the body and need frequent replenishing. They are more difficult to overdose on because the body eliminates them through the urinary tract.

Fat-soluble vitamins are stored in body fat. You still need a regular supply but it can be spread out a bit more. If you lose a great deal of weight, your body will reabsorb the vitamins in the fat and use them.

The vitamins were assigned letters of the alphabet as they were discovered. So vitamin A was the first vitamin discovered, C was the third, E was the fifth, and so on. They were each also given a scientific name. I have included those when they are commonly known, such as vitamin B1, which is called Thiamin.

A and Beta Carotene

(Fat soluble) You need approximately 5,000-50,000$_{IU}$ per day. The body converts Beta Carotene into vitamin A.

Known for being anti-infective and improving night vision. Necessary in bone and teeth development where it forms the connective tissues. Essential to the epithelial cells of the body, a tough sheath of cells that makes up all the covering and linings of the body. The skin is a dry layer of epithelium and the digestive, respiratory and reproductive tracts are lined with it. A is used to protect the body from infections and, in the skin, harmful radiation. It is an antioxidant and renders cancerous cells harmless.

Zinc and protein are required for A to be released into the blood by the liver. E protects A from chemical reactions, helping to make A more available. A helps produce white blood cells.

Processing, cooking and sun drying destroys A and alcohol, iron, mineral oil and cortisone all reduce its absorption.

A is available in yellow-orange and root veggies as well as organ meat. Examples:

Alfalfa Herb	Eggs	Senna Leaf
Barley Grass	Eyebright Herb	Some Squash
Beet Greens	Fish	Spinach
Blessed Thistle	Gotu Kola	Spirulina
Broccoli	Horseradish Root	Stevia Leaf
Cabbage	Liver	Turnips
Cantaloupes	Mangos	Uva Ursi Herb
Capsicum Fruit	Nettle	Yams
(Cayenne	Parsley	Yellow Dock
Pepper)	Peppermint	Root
Carrots	Pumpkins	Yerba Santa
Chaparral Herb	Red Raspberry	
Dandelion Leaf	Leaf	
Dandelion Root	Safflower	

Deficiency (Not enough in your diet) symptoms-

Cataracts	Hearing	microbial
Dry skin	problems	infections
Eye disorders	Increased	Lack of sense of
	susceptibility to	smell or taste

Loss of appetite	Poor nerves	Weight loss
Macular degeneration	Poor night vision	
	Sterility	

Toxicity (too much in your diet) symptoms-

Constipation	Insomnia	Vomiting
Dry skin	Joint pain	
Headaches	Nausea	

Beta carotene is non-toxic, you can't get too much (though if you ate massive amounts of carrots your skin would turn orange).

(The B vitamins were originally thought to be just one vitamin. As it was discovered that they were, in fact, many different vitamins, instead of messing up the naming system, scientists just added numbers to the "B." As they discovered they had misidentified vitamins or that they weren't essential after all, they just eliminated the letter.)

B_1 (Thiamine)

Water soluble, 25-300$_{mg}$ (.33-.5 $_{mg}$ per 1000 kcal of food, minimum of 1mg per day for dieters.)

Helps metabolize carbohydrates. Since it is used up in metabolizing foods and the body doesn't store it, dieters and extreme junk food junkies are in danger of deficiency.

Available in

Acerola fruit	Beans	Burdock root
Asparagus	Beef	Cabbage leaf
Barberry root	Bilberry	Cauliflower
Barley grass	Blue cohosh root	Cereals

Elecampane herb
Enriched pastas
Ephedra
Fenugreek seed
Gotu kola
Grain germs and
brans

Grapevine leaf
Ham
Oranges
Peas
Peppermint
Pork
Rice

Sage leaf
Senna leaf
Spirulina
Wheat germ
Whole grain
breads
Yellow dock root

Deficiency symptoms- mild: appetite and weight loss, nausea, vomiting, fatigue, nervous system problems.

Severe: Beri Beri, muscle weakness, decreased DTR, edema, enlarged heart.

Raw fish and tea contain inhibitors.

Toxicity symptoms-Not generally toxic (You can't eat enough foods to get too much and it would even be difficult to take enough in pill form to cause a problem.)

B$_2$ (Riboflavin)

Water soluble, 25-300$_{mg}$

Helps release energy from carbohydrates, proteins, and fats. Widely distributed in tissues of plants and animals. Helps manufacture red blood cells and corticosteroids. It is not stored in body tissues and must be supplied daily. Can be leached from food while cooking.

Available in

Alfalfa
Asparagus
Barberry Root
Barley Grass
Beans
Blue Cohosh
Root

Broccoli
Cabbage
Capsicum Fruit.
Cauliflower
Cheese
Dairy
Echinacea Root

Ephedra
Eyebright Herb
Fish
Fortified Grains
and Cereals
Gotu Kola
Green Veggies

Hops Flower	Poultry	Yellow Dock
Milk	Spinach	Root
Parsley	Spirulina	Yogurt
Peppermint Leaf	Turnip Greens	

Deficiency symptoms- Mild: cracks and sores to corners of the mouth and tongue, red eyes, skin lesions, dizziness, hair loss, inability to sleep, sensitivity to light, and poor digestion.

Severe: (rare) anemia, nerve disease.

Generally caused by dieters eating non-fortified, refined grains and no dairy products, taking sulfa drugs, oral contraceptives, or exercising vigorously.

Toxicity symptoms- not generally toxic

B_3 (Niacin, nicotinic acid, nicotinamide)

Water-soluble, 25-300 $_{mg}$

An integral part of energy metabolism, facilitates glucose and fat metabolism. Its vasodilating ability (opens up the arteries and blood vessels) can cure tension and migraine headaches. Can reduce cholesterol and prolong blood-clotting time.

Available in

Alfalfa	Cheese	Fish
Asparagus Herb	Chicken Breast	Fortified Breads
Barley Grass	Corn Flour	And Cereals
Beef Liver	Damiana Leaf	Ginkgo
Black Cohosh	Dandelion	Gotu Kola Herb
Brewer's Yeast	Greens	Hops Flower
Broccoli	Dates	Hydrangea Root
Cabbage	Eggs	Milk
Carrots	Eyebright	Mullein
Chamomile	Feverfew	Peanuts

Peppermint Leaf	Red Raspberry Leaf	Tuna
Pork	Slippery Elm Bark	Veal
Potatoes	Spirulina	White Willow Bark
Red Clover Flower	Tomatoes	Whole Grains

Deficiency symptoms- Mild: canker sores, diarrhea, dizziness, fatigue, halitosis, headaches, indigestion, inability to sleep, loss of appetite, dermatitis

Severe: Pellagra (dermatitis, diarrhea, anxiety, depression, irritability)

Toxicity symptoms- nausea, vomiting, abdominal cramps, diarrhea, flushing

Severe: liver damage, irregular heart rate, rash to large portions of the body, gouty arthritis

B$_5$ (Pantothenic acid)

Water soluble, 25-500$_{mg}$

Needed to form coenzyme-A (CoA), and is critical in the metabolism and synthesis of carbohydrates, proteins, and fats.

Available in:

Brewer's Yeast	Liver	Salmon
Fresh Vegetables	Mushrooms	Saltwater Fish
Kidney	Pork	Torula Yeast
Legumes	Royal Jelly	Whole Grains

Deficiency symptoms- rare: nausea, vomiting, fatigue, and headache, tingling in the hands, sleep disturbances, abdominal pains and cramps

Toxicity symptoms- generally not toxic

B$_6$ (Pyridoxine)

Water-soluble, 1.5-2 $_{mg}$

Vitamin B6 processes amino acids, and is also needed to make Serotonin, Melatonin, and Dopamine. Vitamin B6 also aids in the formation of several neurotransmitters, making it an essential nutrient in the regulation of mental processes and possibly mood. Vitamin B_6 lowers homocysteine levels which has been linked to heart disease, stroke, Osteoporosis, and Alzheimer's disease.

A link between vitamin B6 deficiency and carpal tunnel syndrome has been reported in some, but not all, research.

Available in

Avocados	Carrots	Soybeans
Bananas	Chicken	Sunflower
Beef	Eggs	Walnuts
Brewer's Yeast	Oats	Whole Wheat
Brown Rice	Peanuts	

Deficiency symptoms- anemia, seizures, headaches, nausea, dry and flaky skin, sore tongue, cracks on mouth, vomiting

Toxicity symptoms- generally non-toxic, high doses (2000-6000mg/day) can cause nerve disorders.

B_{12} (Cynocobalamin)

Water-soluble, 25-500 $_{mg}$

Structurally the most complicated vitamin. Key in the normal functioning of the brain and nervous system, and for the formation of blood. It is normally involved in the metabolism of every cell of the body, especially affecting DNA synthesis and regulation, but also fatty acid synthesis and energy production.

Historically, vitamin B-12 was discovered from its relationship to the disease Pernicious Anemia, which was eventually discovered to result from an effective lack of this vitamin due to problems with the mechanisms in the body which normally absorb it. Many other subtler kinds of vitamin B_{12} deficiency have since been discovered.

Available in:

All Meats, Dairy	Clams	Lean Beef
Blue Cheese	Cooked Oysters	Liver
Camembert and	Ham	Salmon
Gorgonzola	Herring	Tuna
Cheese	King Crab	

Animal B_{12} is high in absorbable cobalt. Plant B_{12} has a different type of cobalt that is not absorbed by the human body.

Deficiency symptoms-

Chronic fatigue	Headaches	Palpitations
Constipation	Inflammation of	Pernicious
Depression	the tongue	anemia
Digestive	Irritability	Spinal cord
disturbances	Liver	degeneration
Dizziness	enlargement	Tinnitus
Drowsiness	Mood swings	Unsteady gait
Hallucinations	Nerve disorders	

Toxicity symptoms- generally considered non-toxic

C

Water soluble, 60-5000 mg

Speeds wound healing and is an antioxidant. 60mg will prevent scurvy but higher doses are necessary to prevent other illnesses (about 500mg is probably ideal). C is easily lost in processing, so supplementing is often necessary.

Moderates severity of colds and reduces intraocular pressure in Glaucoma, inflammation of Periodontal disease and intolerance to heat.

Can help to concentrate vasodilating prostaglandins to relieve chest tightness in asthmatics.

C is an ingredient of adrenalin and can reduce serum cholesterol and triglycerides. Atherosclerosis can be reduced also. Helps metabolize folic acid and certain amino acids and helps absorb iron. Replaces and strengthens connective tissues. As an antioxidant, it reduces effects of pollution, antibiotics, steroids, oral contraceptives, and smoking.

Available in:

Acerola Fruit
Aloe Vera
Asparagus
Avocados
Barley Grass
Broccoli
Cabbage
Cantaloupe
Cauliflower
Collards
Dandelion
Greens
Hops Flower
Horseradish
Kale

Kiwifruit
Lemons
Lobelia Leaf
Mangos
Onion
Oranges
Papaya
Peppers
Pine Needles
Pineapple
Pink Grapefruit
Potatoes
Pumpkin Seed
Radishes
Raw Fruits

Raw Grass Fed
Milk
Raw Veggies
Red Clover Tops
Red Raspberry
Leaf
Rose Hips
Senna Leaf
Strawberries
Tomatoes
Watercress
Yellow Dock
Root

Deficiency symptoms- mild: poor wound healing, bleeding gums, easy bruising, nosebleeds, joint pain, lack of energy, susceptibility to infection

Severe: scurvy (severe tension, cells fall apart, internal bleeding, death)

Toxicity symptoms-generally considered non-toxic. High doses (5000 mg and up/day) can cause abdominal bloating and diarrhea. Higher doses for long periods of time may contribute to gout.

D

Fat soluble, 400-800$_{IU}$

Vitamin D plays an important role in the maintenance of organ systems. It regulates the calcium and phosphorus levels in the blood, enables normal mineralization of bone, prevents hypocalcemic tetany, affects the immune system by promoting phagocytosis, anti-tumor activity, and immunomodulatory functions. It is also needed for bone growth and bone remodeling by osteoblasts and osteoclasts.

Available in Sunlight (the best source),

Cod Liver Oil	Herring	Sardines
Eggs	Liver	Tuna
Fortified Cereals	Mushrooms	
Fortified Milk	Salmon	

Deficiency symptoms- in infants: irreversible bone deformities.

In children: rickets, delayed tooth development, weak muscles, softened skull

In adults: osteomalcea, osteoporosis, hypocalcaemia

Toxicity symptoms- nausea and vomiting, headaches, constipation, diarrhea, fatigue, loss of appetite, excessive thirst and urination, protein in urine, liver and kidney damage

E

Fat soluble, 30-1200 $_{IU}$

The most important lipid-soluble antioxidant, it protects cell membranes from oxidation, removes the free radical intermediates, protects neurons from damage, and is a cancer prevention.

Available in Vegetable and Nut Oils, Including Soybean, Corn, Safflower, Spinach, Whole Grains, Wheat Germ, and Sunflower Seeds

Deficiency symptoms- rare symptoms may include anemia and edema (swelling).

Toxicity symptoms- generally non-toxic, but stomach upset, dizziness and diarrhea can occur.

K

Fat soluble, 80 $_{mcg}$

Responsible for blood-clotting ability.

Available in Green Leafy Vegetables Including Spinach, Kale, Cauliflower, Broccoli.

Deficiency symptoms- rare except in newborns, where bleeding tendencies are possible, elevated levels of vitamin K can interfere with the effects of anti-coagulants.

Toxicity symptoms- generally non-toxic; but a type of jaundice may occur in premature infants.

Minerals

Minerals are non-organic materials; literally, rocks and dirt. These are necessary for the proper function of the body. Plants absorb them through their roots and we get them through the plants or by eating the animal products and animals that eat the plants.

Calcium

Mineral, 1000-1500 $_{mg}$

Calcium is the main ingredient in bones and teeth; helps regulate blood pressure and the excitability of nerves and the contractility of the muscles and heart. A number of enzymes can't function without it. It helps control blood clotting and is required for absorption of vitamin B_{12}.

Available in:

Asparagus	Crampbark	Oats
Barberry Bark	Damiana Leaf	Pau D' Arco Bark
Broccoli	Figs	Pennyroyal
Buchu Leaf	Grapevine Herb	Plantain
Bupleurum Root	Horsetail Herb	Prunes
Cabbage	Irish Moss	Senna Leaf
Calcium Fortified	Kale	Sesame Seeds
Orange Juice	Kelp	Soybeans
Canned Salmon	Milk (though	Thyme.
And Sardines	highest	Tofu
With The Bones	availability is in	Valerian Root
Still In	raw milk),	Watercress
Carob	Yogurt	Whey
Cheese	Mustard Greens	White Oak Bark
Collard Greens	Nettle Leaf	Wood Betony

Magnesium assists in the absorption of calcium and counters calcium's tendency towards constipation. It should be taken in a ratio of 2:1 Calcium to Magnesium (1000_{mg} calcium: 500_{mg} magnesium).

Potassium aids calcium in controlling blood pressure. Vitamin D aids in the absorption of calcium by the bones as does lactose (milk sugar).

Deficiency symptoms- muscle spasms, rickets, Osteomalacia, Osteoporosis (women are especially prone to deficiency diseases due to pregnancy, nursing and hormones, especially the artificial ones in birth-control pills), high blood pressure.

Sodium causes the body to secret calcium. Phosphorus (found in sodas and processed foods) in too little or too large amounts will also leech calcium. Nitrates will leech calcium from bones. Nitrates are found in processed meats (cold cuts, bacon, sausage, etc) and sodas.

Toxicity symptoms- Hard to get too much, unless your parathyroid glands are overactive, when it can weaken bones, create kidney stones, and interfer with your heart and brain.

Chromium

Trace (needed in teeny, tiny amounts) mineral, 200-600 $_{mg}$

Essential for the production of insulin and cholesterol, it is used in the processing of carbohydrates, especially sugars (which contribute no chromium to the body, so sugar consumption automatically depletes this mineral).

Available in

Barley	Damiana Leaf	Oatstraw
Beer	Dried Beans	Parthenium Root
Brewer's Yeast	Eggs	Peach Bark
Broccoli	Ginkgo	Pollen
Brown Rice	Grape Juice	Potatoes
Buchu Leaf	Gymnema Leaf	Red Clover
Calf's Liver	Ham	Safflower
Catnip	Hibiscus Flower	Spirulina Algae
Cheese	Horseradish Root	Stevia
Chicken	Juniper Berry	Whole Grains
Corn	Lemon Grass	Wine
Corn Oil	Mushrooms	
Dairy Products	Nettle Leaf	

Deficiency symptoms- Alterations in metabolism of fats, carbohydrates, proteins, amino acids. Possibly Hypoglycemia and Diabetes.

Processing foods depletes chromium.

Toxicity symptoms- generally considered non-toxic. Exposure to industrially inhaled chromium has been linked to lung cancer

Copper

Trace mineral, 5_{mg}

Essential to the function of several enzymes, absorption and transport of iron, and the formation of hemoglobin.

Available in:

Avocados	Beans	Brewers Yeast
Barley	Beets	Broccoli

Calf's Liver	Nuts	Seeds
Cocoa Powder	Oats	Shellfish
Gotu Kola Herb	Oranges	Skull Cap
Green Leafy	Pumpkin Seed	White Oak Bark
Vegetables	Radishes	Whole Grains
Horsetail Herb	Raisins	Yucca Root
Lentils	Sage	
Mushrooms	Salmon	

Iron and calcium aid copper absorption.

Deficiency symptoms- Anemia, Osteoporosis, inability of body to manufacture collagen, impaired glucose tolerance, fatigue, baldness, slow growth, slows nervous system development, retardation.

Zinc and copper have an inverse relationship; raising one lowers the other. Ratio should be 5:1 zinc to copper. Fructose, vitamin C, and antacids will prevent the absorption of copper.

Toxicity symptoms- Rare as it is excreted in the urine. Nausea, vomiting, abdominal pain, diarrhea, headaches, metallic taste, hemolytic anemia.

Fluoride

Trace mineral, 1.5-4$_{mg}$

Available in Fluoridated Water, Toothpaste, Tea, Canned Salmon, Mackerel, Kidney, Liver.

Deficiency symptoms- tooth decay, brittle bones.

Toxicity symptoms- mottled teeth, osteomalacia, and osteoporosis.

Some believe we are getting way too much fluoride between water fluoridation and modern toothpastes. This is a toxic chemical and can kill if too much is ingested (thus the warning on toothpaste tubes to not let children ingest it).

Many also believe the research showing the benefits of fluoride to the teeth were poorly done and biased towards industries that needed a way to dispose of this toxic chemical.

I don't know the truth, really. But since most if not all of our food is grown and processed in fluoridated water, the chances are you could use a non-fluoride toothpaste (or plain ole' baking soda) without damage and lower your risks of toxicity.

Folic acid

Water soluble, 400-1200 $_{mcg}$

Needed for DNA synthesis, preventing neural tube birth defects as well as other birth defects. It also appears to protect against cleft palate and cleft lip formation. It is needed to make chemicals which affect moods and control amino acid levels in the blood. This lowers the risk of heart disease, osteoporosis, strokes, and Alzheimer's disease.

Available in:

Asparagus	Dates	Navy Beans
Barley	Fortified Cereals	Okra
Beef	Green Leafy	Oranges
Bran	Vegetables	Pinto Beans
Brewer's Yeast	Lamb	Pork
Broccoli	Legumes	Spinach
Brown Rice	Lentils	Split Peas
Brussels Sprouts	Liver	Tuna
Cheese	Milk	Whole Grains
Chicken	Mushrooms	

Deficiency symptoms- anemia, irritability, weakness, sleep disturbances, pallor, sore and reddened tongue.

Toxicity symptoms- generally considered non-toxic.

Iodine

Mineral, 0-150 $_{mcg}$ (most individuals) 150-300 $_{mcg}$ (for those living in low iodine areas or for those with low iodine diets.)

A trace mineral needed to make thyroid hormones, which are necessary for maintaining normal metabolism in all cells of the body.

Available in Iodized Salt, Shellfish, Saltwater Fish, Milk, and Seaweed.

Deficiency symptoms- growth and sexual development can be delayed in children, Goiter (swelling of the thyroid).

Question: since all of our salt has iodine added to it and everything we eat is salted, why is everyone in our country on thyroid medicine? The answer is that, though we ingest plenty of iodine, we destroy it by eating sugar and white flour and not exercising enough. Thus, we all have malfunctioning thyroids.

Toxicity symptoms- generally considered non-toxic if under 1000 mcg/day. High doses can cause headaches, metallic taste in mouth and rash. Doses over 20,000 mcg/day have been associated with Iodide Goiter.

Iron

Mineral, 15-25$_{mg}$ (men), 18-30 $_{mg}$ (women) (You need to consume approximately 1000 calories to get 6$_{mg}$ of iron. Thus a woman would need 3000 calories per day to get enough iron. Most American women need no more than 2000 calories to maintain their weight. This is why anemia in Americans is so common.)

A constituent of hemoglobin and myoglobin, iron aids in the transport of oxygen to the cells and carbon dioxide to the lungs. Many enzymes require iron to help attack microbes in the blood.

Available in:

Althea Root	Dandelion Root	Mullein
Avocados	Dates	Nuts
Baked Potatoes	Devil's Claw Root	Peaches
Barberry	Dried Prunes	Pears
Beef	Eggs	Pennyroyal
Beets	Fish	Pumpkin Seeds
Bilberry	Green Leafy	Raisins
Blue Cohosh	Vegetables	Red Raspberry
Brewer's Yeast	Horsetail Herb	Leaf
Bucher's Broom	Iron Fortified	Sesame Seeds
Burdock	Cereals	Soybeans
Catnip	Kelp	Thyme
Celery Seed	Lentils	Uva Ursi
Chickweed	Liver	Whole Grains
Clams	Milk Thistle	Yerba Santa

Iron from meats absorb easier than from plants, though it is in leafy greens.

You can also raise your iron consumption by cooking in cast iron pots and pans. Trace amounts of the mineral leach into your food.

Vitamin C, citric acid, fructose found in honey and amino acids derived from proteins aid absorption.

Deficiency symptoms-

Anemia	Dizziness	Nervousness
Coarse hair	Dry	Pallor
Cracked lips or tongue	Dysphasia	Sleepiness
Depression.	Fatigue	Slowed mental
	Hair loss	response

Tannic acids, phosphates, milk, cheese, sodas, alcohol, and aspirin hinder its absorption- coffee and tea by as much as 50% (because of tannin content). Calcium, magnesium, zinc, copper, manganese and cadmium also interfere with iron absorption.

Toxicity symptoms- generally considered non-toxic if under 75 mg/day. High doses can cause abdominal cramps, vomiting, and diarrhea. Severe overdoses of iron can be considered fatal if medical attention is not sought.

Magnesium

Mineral, 500-750 mg. We get approximately 120 mg per 1000 calories of food.

Vital to the synthesis of RNA, DNA and proteins. Essential in the metabolism of proteins, carbohydrates and lipids. Over 300 enzymes require the presence of magnesium to function including alkaline phosphatase which is used to activate calcium and phosphorus metabolism.

It regulates muscle contraction and helps in the utilization of vitamins B_6, C and E. The brain stores twice as much as other body tissues.

Available in:

Althea root
Apples
Apricots
Astragalus root
Avocados
Baked potatoes
Bananas
Boneset herb
Brewer's yeast
Broccoli
Brown rice
Bupleurum root
Burdock root
Cantaloupes
Chickweed

Devil's claw root
Dog grass
Dulse herb
Elecampane root
Grapefruit
Haddock
Humeric seed
Irish moss
Kelp
Leafy greens
Lemons
Licorice root
Lima beans
Navy beans
Nettle leaf

Nuts
Oatmeal
Oatstraw
Pennyroyal
Peppermint leaf
Pumpkin seed
Salmon
Senna leaf
Sesame seeds
Siberian ginseng
Spinach
Tofu
Wheat
White willow bark
Yogurt

Vitamin D and calcium are essential for absorption.
Deficiency symptoms- widespread- an estimated 70-80% of Americans are deficient. Processed foods are probably the biggest cause. Those who drink "soft water" do not get enough.

Headaches
Angina pain
Arrhythmias of
the heart
Calcium oxalate
kidney stone
formation
Confusion

Congestive heart
failure
Constipation
Craving for
sweets
Sleep
disturbances
Epilepsy and
migraines

Gi upset
High ldl
Hypertension
Irritability
Kwashiorkor
Muscle spasms
Rapid heartbeat
Strokes
Thrombosis

Chronic deficiency is caused by diuretics, digitalis, antibiotics, chemotherapy, alcohol and excessive fats or protein intake, and stress.

Sodium, saturated fat, excess protein, calcium, potassium, phosphorus, and lactose hinder magnesium's work.

Toxicity symptoms- Rarely toxic. Symptoms may include diarrhea, fatigue, depression, and arrhythmia.

Manganese

Trace mineral, 15-30 $_{mg}$

Required by the body to produce healthy connective tissues like cartilage. A cofactor in enzymes that transfer phosphate groups and thus an important factor in energy metabolism. Can raise your HDL levels and strengthens your immune system.

Available in all plant tissues but especially in leaves and seeds;

Apples	Figs	Salmon
Apricots	Ginger Root	Seeds
Avocados	Gotu Kola Herb	Shellfish
Bananas	Grapefruit	Soybeans
Bilberry	Grapevine Herb	Spirulina
Blue Cohosh	Green Leafy	Tea
Brewer's Yeast	Vegetables	Tofu
Buchu Leaf	Hibiscus Flower	Uva Ursi Leaf
Canned	Hydrangea Root	Wheat Bran
Pineapple Juice	Lady's Slipper	Wheat Germ
Cantaloupe	Herb	White Oak Bark
Catnip	Milk Thistle Herb	Whole Grains
Chickweed	Nuts	Wood Betony
Cocoa	Peaches	Herb
Dairy Products	Red Raspberry	Yerba Santa
Dog Grass	Leaf	

Deficiency symptoms- rare:

And hearing
Arteriosclerosis
Confusion
Elevated
cholesterol levels
Grinding of teeth
Impaired vision

Increased blood
pressure
Increased heart
rate
Irritability
Mental
impairment

Pancreatic
damage
Skin rash
Sweating
Tremors

Toxicity symptoms- generally considered non-toxic. Exposure to industrially inhaled manganese has been linked to psychiatric and nervous disorders.

Molybdenum

Trace mineral, 75_{mcg}

An essential trace mineral needed for certain enzyme-dependent processes, including the metabolism of iron.

Preliminary evidence indicates that molybdenum, through its involvement in detoxifying sulfites, might reduce the risk of sulfite-reactive asthma attacks.

Available in:

Beans
Cereals
Dark Green
Leafy Vegetables

Legumes
Meats
Milk Products
Peas

Whole Grains

Deficiency symptoms- rare: increased heart rate, mouth and gum disorders, impotence in older males, increased respiratory rate, night blindness.

Toxicity symptoms- generally considered non-toxic.

Phosphorus

Mineral, 1200_{mg}
Makes up much of the skeletal system,
Available in:

Asparagus	Extra Lean	Peppermint
Barley Grass	Ground Beef	Pumpkin
Bilberry	Fennel Seed	Salmon
Blue Cohosh	Ginkgo Leaf	Sesame Seed
Broccoli	Halibut	Siberian Ginseng
Buchu Leaf	Highly	Root
Cabbage Herb	Carbonated	Soybean
Cauliflower Herb	Beverages	Sunflower Seeds
Chicken Breast	Horseradish Root	Yellow Dock
Corn	Legumes	Root
Cranberry	Lima Beans	Yerba Santa
Dairy Products	Milk	Herb
Dog Grass	Milk Thistle Seed	Yogurt
Dried Fruits	Nuts	
Eggs	Oatmeal	

Can decrease absorption of other minerals
Deficiency symptoms- extremely unlikely; fatigue, irritability, decreased appetite, bone pain, weakness, skin sensitivity.
Toxicity symptoms- rarely toxic. Symptoms may include brittle bones related to loss of calcium (osteoporosis). Since it is contained in sodas, this is becoming more common.

Potassium

Trace mineral, 2.5 grams (1:1 ratio with sodium)

Crucial to osmotic equilibrium, the way which cells are nourished and cleansed. The principle catalyst in intracellular fluids and helps cells maintain volume, assists in carbohydrate metabolism, protein synthesis, muscle contraction and nerve impulse conduction,

Available in:

Asparagus	Cauliflower	Hydrangea Root
Baked Potatoes	Celery	Lemon Grass
Barley Grass	Dulse Herb	Parsley
Blessed Thistle	Feverfew	Peppermint
Broccoli	Fruits	Raw Plants
Bupleurum Root	Grains	Veggies
Cabbage	Dried Apricots	Sage
Carrot	Hops	Skullcap
Catnip	Horseradish	

Sodium antagonist.

Deficiency symptoms-

Acne	Edema	Impaired
Arrhythmia	Elevated	cognitive function
Chills	cholesterol	Increased blood
Decreased reflex	Glucose	pressure
response	intolerance	Insomnia
Diarrhea	Growth	Muscle spasms
Dry skin	retardation	Thirst

Toxicity symptoms- rarely toxic. Symptoms may include arrhythmia and heart failure (doses exceeding 18gm/day).

Selenium

Mineral, 100-400 $_{mcg}$ (those living in low-selenium areas such as costal and glaciated regions) 50-200 $_{mcg}$ (those living in high selenium areas)

Selenium is an anti-oxidant, the same as vitamin E. It can replace sulfur in certain amino acids. Highly concentrated in the pancreas, pituitary, and liver. Supplementation can strengthen the immune system by increasing antibody production. Low selenium is correlated with heart disease though we don't yet know why.

Available in:

Althea root	Dairy products	Pumpkin seed
Barberry root	Dog grass	Salmon
Bayberry root	Dulse herb	Sarsaparilla root
Black cohosh root	Hibiscus flower	Shellfish
	Ho shou wu root	Torula yeast
Blessed thistle herb	Lady's slipper herb	Tuna
Blue cohosh root	Lemon grass	Valerian root
Brazil nuts	Lobster	Vegetables
Broccoli	Milk thistle seed	Wheat germ
Brown rice	Onions	Wheat grains
Buchu leaf	Organ meats	Whole grains
Catnip herb	Poultry	Yarrow flower
		Yerba santa herb

Deficiency symptoms- muscle weakness, linked to cancer and heart disease, fatigue, growth retardation, elevated, cholesterol levels, susceptibility to infection, sterility, irritability, nail, hair and tooth damage.

Toxicity symptoms-rarely toxic. Symptoms may include garlic breath, brittle hair and nails, irritability, liver and kidney impairment, metallic taste in mouth, dermatitis, and jaundice.

Sodium

Trace mineral, 2400 mg (average daily intake in America is 5000-10,000mg)

Keeps the fluid in the body at the right proportion inside and outside the cells. Helps transmit nerve impulses as an electrolyte.

Available in:

Barley grass	Cheese	Oatstraw
Bread	Comfrey root	Parsley
Buchu leaf	Gotu kola	Pennyroyal herb
Cabbage	Grapefruit	Peppermint leaf
Canned soups	Licorice root	Rose hips
Canned tuna	Milk	Safflowers
Canned vegetables	Most anything processed	Sardines
Carrot	Most meats	Sea food
Celery herb	especially ham	Seaweed
Cereals	and bacon	Wild yam root
Chamomile		

Deficiency symptoms- rare in America;

Abdominal cramps	Fatigue	Palpitations
Confusion	Headaches	Seizures.
Dehydration	Impaired taste	Vomiting
Depression	Low blood pressure	
Dizziness	Nausea	

Toxicity symptoms-edema, elevated blood pressure, potassium deficiency, diseases of the liver and kidney.

Silicon

Abundant inorganic element, major component of sand and glass, good semiconductor, helps give strength to bones. Good for the hair and nails.

Available in:

Astragals root	Echinacea root	Lady's slipper
Burdock root	Eyebright herb	herb
Butcher's broom	Ginger root	Lemon grass
root	Golden seal root	Licorice
Chickweed	Gotu kola	Oatstraw herb
Corn silk	Horsetail herb	Thyme herb
Dog grass	Hydrangea root	Turmeric seed
Dulse herb		

Zinc

Mineral, 15-50 $_{mg}$. Average intake is half

Important for healthy skin and nails, proper wound healing, successful pregnancies, male virility and sense of taste. It strengthens the membranes of the body, including the heart, making them less susceptible to injury, acts as an anti-oxidant, and strengthens the immune system.

Available in:

Astragalus root	Elecapane herb	Mushrooms
Beef	Fish	Nettle leaf
Bilberry	Irish moss herb	Nuts
Buchu leaf	Lady's slipper	Parthenium root
Capsicum fruit	herb	Pecans
Chickweed herb	Lamb	Pennyroyal
Cooked oysters	Legumes	Poultry
Dulse herb	Lima beans	Pumpkin and
Echinacea root	Liver	sunflower seeds
Eggs	Mistletoe herb	Sage leaf

Sardines	Soybeans	Wild yam root
Scullcap herb	Spirulina	Yogurt
Siberian ginseng	Whole grains	

Deficiency symptoms- change in taste and smell, nails can become brittle and peel, acne, delayed sexual maturation, hair lose, elevated cholesterol, impaired night vision, impotence, growth retardation, increased susceptibility to infection.

Defecincy can impair newborns immune system. May be linked to cancer.

Topical aplication on throats reduces colds by seven days on average.

Toxicity symptoms- nausea, vomiting, abdominal pain, impaired coordination, fatigue.

Other nutrients

Probiotics

Bacteria in dirt that helps us digest our food. Some digestive troubles today may be linked to too clean of a food supply. Available in pills and live-culture yogurt, kefir, and other fermented foods.

Digestive enzymes

Chemical catalysts that help to dissolve our food.

Both of the above are available in pill form. Some say they help. Some say they are a hoax. Do your research and decide for yourself.

Appendex B- Body Systems

There are 10 systems to the human body and it helps to understand them and how they work when we are trying to be healthy.

➤ The **Respiratory System** – Also called "breathing." Respiration is taking oxygen and other, more minor gasses into the body, and sending the toxic Carbon Dioxide out of the body.

Your lungs are protected by your ribcage. You breathe in by contracting your diaphragm, a flat muscle underneath your lungs, just at the rib level. This causes the chest to expand, drawing air in.

As you take air into your lungs, the oxygen is added to the blood circulating through the 6 million tiny air sacks inside your lungs called "alveoli" which are covered in capillaries, and are the smaller parts of the bronchus. This all looks kind of like a bunch of grapes inside two bags (your lungs).

At the same time the oxygen is added to the blood, the Carbon Dioxide is taken out. This is one way your body gets rid of toxins. Good air in- bad air out.

The respiratory system runs from the nose and mouth to the lungs. You keep this system healthy by:

o Avoiding pollution of all kinds as much as possible. This means **DON'T SMOKE!** And don't live with someone who does. (See the chapter on Air) Smoking is the major cause of lung cancer, though big city air can be nearly as bad.

o Exercising so all those tiny little bags expand and contract, to keep these muscles limber and flexible.

- o Wash your hands regularly to prevent infections
- o Eat a **healthy, vitamin-rich diet**
- o Drink plenty of water
- o Introduce plants into your living spaces, as well as other air-cleaning measures.

➢ **The Digestive System/Excretory System** – This system includes the mouth, throat, stomach, and intestines.

Food (fuel for the human being) is taken into the mouth, and reduced in size to manageable bits, while adding saliva, which chemically breaks nutrients down to microscopic levels.

It then moves through the throat to the stomach where it is mixed with more digestive fluids to further break it down.

This goopy mixture is then slowly sent to the small intestines where nutrients are absorbed into the body. From there is goes to the large intestines where more is taken out and the rest is sent to the toilet.

Keep your digestive system functioning great by:

- o Eating lots of fiber (a grown woman needs around 25 grams a day, a man 35- that's fruit, veggies, beans, and whole grains)
- o Exercising. We are designed to move.
- o Drinking lots of water.
- o Brush your teeth at least once a day. If you teeth are bad you can't chew, which reduces your chances of getting the nutirents you need. In addition, the bacteria left on your teeth, especially after eating sugar, can travel to the rest of your body and make you sick.
- o Eat probiotics (i.e. yogurt, most fermented foods)

- o Keep a fairly regular eating schedule. Your body likes to know when its next meal will be.
- o Keep stress under control. Messes the tummy up.
- ➤ **Cardiovascular/Circulatory System** – This is your blood system and is kind of like the freeway of your body. Blood carries nutrients to all your cells, and waste products away from them, as well as carrying disease fighting white blood cells.

This system includes your heart, arteries (carrying oxygen and nutrients), and veins (which carry your waste products). The heart pumps the fluid around and around.

Keep this system healthy with:
- o Exercise. Make your heart beat faster for roughly 15 minutes a day.
- o Avoiding refined sugars as much as possible.
- o Avoiding man-made fats (margarine, Crisco)
- o Avoiding stress
- o Avoid smoking and alcohol, as well as excess caffeine.
- o Eat a nutrient rich diet.
- ➤ **Renal System/Urinary System** – This system includes the kidneys and bladder and filters liquid waste products out of your blood, taking them away (through your pee). Keep this system healthy by:
- o Drinking lots of water.
- o Limit alcohol and caffeine.
- o Don't smoke.
- o Exercise.
- o Eat lots of fiber.

- o Do pelvic floor muscle (Kegel) exercises. At least once a day squeeze the muscles that stop pee when you are sitting on the toilet.
- o Use the bathroom often and when needed. Holding urine in your bladder for too long can weaken your bladder muscles and make a bladder infection more likely.
- o Take enough time to fully empty the bladder when urinating. Rushing may not allow you to fully empty the bladder, which will increase your risk of infection.
- o Wipe from front to back after using the toilet. This keeps bacteria from getting into the urethra. This step is most important after a bowel movement.
- o Wear cotton underwear and loose-fitting clothes. Wearing loose, cotton clothing will allow air to keep the area around the urethra dry. Tight-fitting jeans and nylon underwear can trap moisture and help bacteria grow.

➢ **Endocrine System** – "Endocrine" is a fancy way of saying "hormones and chemical signals." This system includes the pineal gland, pituitary gland (in the brain), thyroid (in the neck just under the jaw), adrenal glands, pancreas, and ovaries (if you are female) and testes (if you are male).

Hundreds of hormones tell your cells and organs what to do. They help control things like your appetite and your blood pressure, and how your body reacts to stress. An example is the way insulin tells your cells how to use sugar for energy. Sex hormones control male and female traits, puberty, fertility, childbirth, and menopause.

Keep this system healthy by:

- Exercise, drink water, eat fiber
- Make sure you get enough iodine (for your thyroid)
- Get plenty of sunshine (increases the hormone serotonin, which helps sleep, mood, and depression, as well as vitamin D which helps your immune system among other things.)
- If you can afford it, eat organic, grassfed foods.
- Avoid chemical estrogen mimics (cleaners, air fresheners, pesticides.) This would also include chemical birth controls.
- Limit junk food (including alcohol, caffeine, and anything made in a factory) Gums up the works and confuses your body.
- Get plenty of sleep. Exahstion disrupts your hormones.

➤ **<u>Nervous System</u>** – Including your brain and nerves, this it the communication system in your body. All five of your senses function through your nerves: sight, hearing, taste, touch, and smell, as well as our thoughts, emotions, and reflexes. Keep this system healthy by:

- Eating well (especially B_{12}, D, and healthy fats such as butter and cocoanut oil).
- Don't smoke or drink to excess.
- Have a regular sleep schedule.
- Exercise you mind by playing mind games (i.e. Sudoco, Crosswords), and writing with a pen and paper, doing things with your left hand you normally do with your right (like driving or sweeping the floor).
- Exercise the rest of your body (increases blood flow which helps clean toxins out of your brain

- o Avoid toxic chemicals and too many repetitive motion activities (i.e. spending 8 hours a day every day for years crocheting).
- o Pray. Settles you, centers you.
- o Go for a walk without shoes. This is believed to help dispurse positive ions and generally improve your health in many ways. Walking barefoot can further help by improving your sleep and strengthening your immune system. It has been accredited with reducing pain and inflammation, reducing the risk of heart disease, normalizing biological rhythms, increasing your senses, improving overall posture, lessens the severity of menstrual cramps.
- o Having a cup of Green Tea at least once a day, is a great way of maintaining the heart of your nervous system. Rich in amino acid, Green Tea helps with serotonin levels. Besides, caffeine in green tea aids in increasing concentration, thinking ability and focusing. It is also a great way of treating insomnia, diabetes and Parkinson's disease.
- o Drink plenty of water.
- o Consume adaptogenic herbs (such as astrologis).

➤ **Musculoskeletal system** – Your muscles and bones, as well as the ligaments and cartlege that holds them together. Gives your body structure and shape and allows you to move around. Keep this system healthy with:

- o Regular exercise, especially weight-bearing exercise. Aim for an hour a day, most days. Carrying weights makes your bones stronger and thicker.
- o Don't overextend your joints. Pain is a warning. ("Aches" are not pain.)
- o Eat a variety of …oh you know, the same things for everything else, especially high calcium foods.
- o Get plenty of D, preferably through sunlight.
- o Don't smoke or drink to excess. This has been shown to weaken bones. As does too many sodas.
- o Wear protective gear when possible (such as seatbelts and helmets.)
- ➢ **Integumentary System/Exocrine System** – What people see; your skin, hair, nails, and sweat glands. These protect your body from germs and injury,and regulate its temperature and moisture content.
  - o Get some sunlight, but not too much. Burning does long term damage as well as hurting in the short term.
  - o Don't smoke.
  - o Limit bath time and temperature. Hot water and long showers or baths remove oils from your skin. Bathing removes oils from your skin, and you can burn yourself with too hot shower water. However…
  - o Bathe regularly and wash your hands regularly. Keeps your skin and nails clean to prevent infections.

- Occasionally scrub your skin with something rough (like a brush or soft scrub sponge). This encourages circulation and removes dead skin cells.
- Cut your fingernails and toenails straight across after bathing to avoid hangnails. Occasional soaking in soapy water or rubbing cocoanut oil into your nails helps them stay in good condition.
- Avoid strong soaps, shampoos, and chemicals.
- Occasionally soak your hair with a warmed oil (olive or cocoanut are good) and wrap with a warm towel. This improves hair texture, shine, and overall health.
- Shave carefully. To protect and lubricate your skin, apply shaving cream, lotion or gel (or a good layer of soap bubbles) before shaving. For the closest shave, use a clean, sharp razor. Shave in the direction the hair grows, not against it.
- Pat dry. After washing or bathing, gently pat or blot your skin dry with a towel so that some moisture remains on your skin.
- Moisturize dry skin. If your skin is dry, use a moisturizer that fits your skin type. Some prefer pure cocoanut oil because of its lack of bad chemicals and the presence of good "fat" vitamins. (Drinking lots of water will also help your skin stay moist.)
- Eat a healthy diet high in green leafies, and don't stress. Nettle Leaf and Shave Grass are known to be especially good for your hair and nails.

➢ **Lymphatic System/Immune System** – This system includes the lymph nodes, white blood cells, T cells, spleen, thymus gland, tonsils (which filter bacteria out of your food as you eat it), and adenoids (located at the back of your nose to filter the air you breath and your food). There are lymph nodes in your body that you can likely feel under your arm (in your armpit), in each groin (at the top of your legs) and in your neck. There are also lymph nodes you may not be able to feel, such as those found in your abdomen, pelvis and chest.

Lymph fluid travels through its own capillaries that are much smaller than veins. This system circulates only by gravity and movement (including deep breathing). It has no heart to pump it through your body, like the circulatory system does.

Lymphatic fluid cleans up waste and returns it to the blood. As this fluid passes through lymph nodes the white blood cells, which are made in the nodes, attack invaders (germs) and kill them.

Cancer often breaks away from the original tumor and gets caught in the nodes. This is why doctors check the nodes when they are checking for cancer.

A build up of lymphatic fluid is a sign of injury or toxic invaders. This is inflammation and causes pain.

The spleen filters blood, removing old red blood cells and replacing them with new red blood cells that are made in the bone marrow.

The lymphatic system also helps to remove garbage from the body, such as carbon dioxide and the byproducts of cellular feeding on oxygen, minerals and nutrients. This system helps to remove these impurities and dispose of them through perspiration, bowel movements, urine and your breath.

The lymphatic system helps defend the body against illness-causing germs, bacteria, viruses and fungi by making special white blood cells (called lymphocytes) that produce antibodies which are responsible for immune responses that defend the body against disease.
You keep it strong and health by:

- o Eat healthy (especially leafy greens, the cabbage family, nuts and seeds, fish, berries, olive oil, cocoanut oil, ginger, garlic, turmeric, burdock, milk thistle, and similar herbs), exercise, drink lots of water, get enough sleep.
- o Get a massage. Actually, you can do most of a massage on yourself by simply rubbing each part of your skin and muscles gently but firmly. This increases the circulation of lymphatic fluid, carrying away toxins and bringing in nutrients and white blood cells. It also reduces inflammatory tissues, relieving pain.
- o Shake it up. Bounceing helps the lymphatic fluids to move around more, so jog, bounce on a trampoline, dance, etc. Even something as gentle as yoga helps.
- o Don't wear clothes (including bras) that are too tight. This restricts the flow of lymph fluid.
- o Keep your gut healthy by eating fermented foods and fish (which has omega 3's).
- o Nettle leaf helps the body heal from allergies, and many herbs help strengthen the immune system. Almost all essential oils, garlic, ginger, and "hot" herbs will help kill germs.

- The fewer toxins your body is exposed to the less work your lymphatic system has to do and the more it can "focus" on taking out normal waste and real invaders. So reduce the toxins you are exposed to as much as possible.

However, we live in a world where you can't remove everything bad. God did make our bodies powerful enough to take care of a lot of baddies with no side affects. So, avoid the bads you can, but don't stress about the ones you can't

- Pray. The quiet, peace, and breathing that goes with prayer helps strengthen the entire immune system.

➢ **Reproductive System** – In females, this includes the breasts, ovaries, uterus, vagina, and vulva. In males, the penis and testes. These organs are involved in reproduction- creating new human beings, as well as hormone production and regulation mentioned above systems.

Keep your reproductive system healthy by:
- The as same as with everything else: eat a good, healthy diet, exercise, drink plenty of water, get plenty of rest.
- Avoid tabacco, too much alcohol and cafeene, and stress.
- Regular bathing to prevent infection.
- Do not have sex until you marry. There are a number of diseases that can be transferred through sex and the best way to avoid them is to not have sex except inside of marriage. If you do decide to have sex outside of marriage, use a condom. It offers some protection against disease.

- For males, wear a protective cup when playing contact sports. Injury to the reproductive organs, besides being painful, can result in infertility.
- If you are a girl and use tampons, be sure to change them every four to six hours. Leaving tampons in for too long can put you at risk of Toxic Shock Syndrome. This is a serious condition. Signs and symptoms of Toxic Shock Syndrome develop suddenly, and the disease can be fatal. Symptoms are fever, shock, and problems with the function of several body organs.
- Women should also get in the habit of doing a monthly self-exam to check for breast cancer. Breast cancer is rare in teens, but it's a good idea to start doing the exam when you are young to build the habit and help you get to know what is normal for you.
- Chemical birth controls mess up your sytem so it doesn't know how it's supposed to act. Estrogen in "The Pill" acts by making your body think it is already pregnant, and so most of the time you won't ovulate (send a mature egg out to be fertilized). Sometimes, though, an egg goes out anyway, so "The Pill" also contains progesterone that makes your uterus inhabitable to a fertilized egg, which simply passes out in the period.
- Each full term baby a woman has sends fetal stem cells throughout her system during pregnancy. These cells adapt to help some systems that may be malfunctioning. So, each full term baby a woman has lowers her risk of cancer- especially reproductive cancers- by 2%.

- Breast feeding casues a woman's body to produce oxytocin which causes the uterus to contract (kind of like exercising without the sweat). This helps the uterus to return to nomal size after birth. (Oxytocin, by the way, also casuses you to fall in love. Men produce it in large amounts after orgasim and women when cuddling. It also strengthens the heart, helping to protect against heart disease).
- Breast feeding has also been shown to reduce the insedence of breast cancer by 7% for every year spent nursing (one Asian country has the custom of only every breast feeding on the right side. It is considered rude and low class to nurse on both sides. In this nation, women never get breast cancer in the right breast but frequently do in the left.)
- Keep track of your cycles, your moods during the month, and generally how you feel. This will give you clues to what herbal supplements you may need as well as when you are fertile (women are only actually fertile 3-10 days a month.)
- 1-3 cups of raspberry tea a day is great for a woman's reproductive system. This herb helps regulate periods, reduce the risk of miscarriage, help a miscarriage complete faster if it is inevitable (the baby too malformed to live), reduces the risk of early labor, helps contractions in labor be strong and regular, reduces bleeding with birth, and encourages milk production.
- Play. This is good for all of your systems and health. It means frequent sex after you marry, too.
- Get a pap smear (a test where the doctor inserts a swab into the vagina and then sends it to a lab to test for cancer) every 3-5 years.

- Get a mammogram (a special x-ray that looks for abnormalities inside the breasts), ummm, well, look it up? There is disagreement on the the time to start and frequency. Some say to get your first one at 40 and every year after that until age 55, then every other year until 74. Others say the first one should be at 45, while others say 50 unless you have other factors predisposing you to breast cancer (like a close relative who has had it.) Nearly everyone says after 74 any cancers that are there will grow too slowly to affect the lifespan of the woman, so you can quit bothering then. Since this issue is so up in the air, see what the current guidelines are and talk to your doctor. (There is currently some testing going on to accomplish the same thing as a mammogram by having the woman wear a special sports bra for 24 hours. This bra has electronic sensors that build a picture of the breast without the radiation of a mammogram. The doctor simply plugs the bra's usb into a computer and sees what's going on.)

I, personally, waited until I was 50 for my first one. I haven't yet decided whether I will do this once a year of every other year. This was a decision I actually made when considering all my risk factors, but before my own mother was diagnosed with breast cancer. I decided not to change my plans after her diagnosis, but many would disagree with my decision. At this point, no harm done, but I don't know that I would recommend someone else to follow the same course. Certainly, pray about it and look at the most recent research.

- Do not get an abortion. They are clearly linked to breast cancer, increase your risk of infertility, as well as miscarriages, and mental illness. That's besides the moral issues.

- Women quit having periods and being able to have children at around age 50. This is called "menopause." The body does a lot of changing around this time, but the basic recommendations for health are the same: exercise, good foor, play, trust God. Evening Primrose Oil and progesterone cream made from wild yam help with the symptoms (hot flashes, dry skin, etc).

Recommended reading

What the Bible Says About Healthy Living *by Dr Rex Russell.* Dr Russell compared studies on nutrition and health with the Bible to come up with some interesting correlations.

Nourishing traditions *by Sally Fallon.* A great deal of information on natural eating plus a telephone-book-sized cookbook.

Real Food *by Nina Planck.* A book outlining the benefits of a natural diet.

Eat This Not That *by David Zinczenko.* Mr. Zinczenko was once "The Fat Kid." Through nutrition information and wise choices he reshaped his body. He shares that information with us through this series of books. He breaks down the nutrition of each product and compares it with other similar products to discover what the healthiest choices are (i.e. Which is healthier; McDonald's Quarter Pounder, Wendy's Single, or Carl's Jr's Famous Star?).

The Eating Better Cookbooks *by Sue Gregg.* Mrs. Gregg, a dietician and a Christian, has come up with many delicious, inexpensive, healthy recipes. These books are devided by meals and written with the idea of using them as textbooks to teach cooking.

Naturally Healthy Woman, Naturally Healthy Pregnancy, Mommy Diagnostics, Naturally Healthy Cuisine *By Shonda Parker.* Mrs. Parker is a professional, Christian herbalist. Her advise is balanced and thoroughly none "New Age-Y."

What Your Doctor May Not be Telling You About Menopause and **What your Doctor May Not be Telling You About Peri-Menopause** *by Dr John Lee.* Dr Lee's research shows that progesterone/estrogen imbalance is the cause of many problems suffered by many women. Progesterone can be changed in the body to whatever hormone is needed.

Any book by Larry Burkett. Mr. Burkett was the first Christian financial advisor. His advice has helped many to reorganize their finances and get out of debt.

Financially Challenged *by Wilson J. Humber* My favorite financial book.

Rich Dad Poor Dad Wise advice from a man who learned valuble lessons from two different men in his life.

What your doctor may not be telling you about vaccines. More vaccine information.

Soulful Simplicity The author was diagnosed with MS which led to her discovering a better way to live. Very valuble advise for surviving in today's world.

www.ingramcontent.com/pod-product-compliance
Lightning Source LLC
Chambersburg PA
CBHW031506270326
41930CB00006B/269